Don't Sweat It! Manage Your Menopause In 21 Days

Ailsa Petchey

Amazon

Published by Amazon

.

ISBN 9798538238286

Any medical references, questionnaire results, documentation used in the book can be found under references at the back of the book.

Front cover illustration: Jacqueline Bissett

Front cover & book design: Katherine McAdam, Brand Magic Printed by Amazon, in the United Kingdom

First Printing edition 2021.

AilsaPetchey

3 High Street, Woburn Sands, Milton Keynes MK17 8RQ

www.50shadesofenopause.co.uk

Typesetting services by BOOKOW.COM

This book is dedicated to my amazing long suffering husband Michael and children Callum and Ella who are my world and make sense of the madness!

To my sister, mother and all the amazing women I've met, worked and shared time with – your support, laughter, tears and strength are a daily inspiration.

Preface

'If you focus on results, you won't see the change, but if you focus on the change, you'll see results!'

Going through menopause? Then this book is for you!

My daily mantra is 'you've totally got this!' and with this book and programme you have totally got the support, encouragement and knowledge you need to succeed in getting you through menopause without the struggle.

This book is for all women entering menopause whatever your age or stage. You maybe in the early stage of perimenopause dealing with the myriad of symptoms that have come at you from out of the blue. Or you might be in post menopause, where you're years past your final period, but things still just don't feel right and the fatigue, body aches, hot sweats are still bothering you!

Just know that this is a step-by-step guide to help ease your symptoms, find hormonal balance and work out what you need to do to maintain equilibrium as you continue through your life, in a simple easy to follow 21 day programme.

Learn about menopause and take action provided in the book and on the website to see the changes you want.

Let's go!

Acknowledgments

A big thank you to

Jacqueline Bissett for my book cover illustration

&

Katherine McAdam at Brand Magic for

the book design & website

Contents

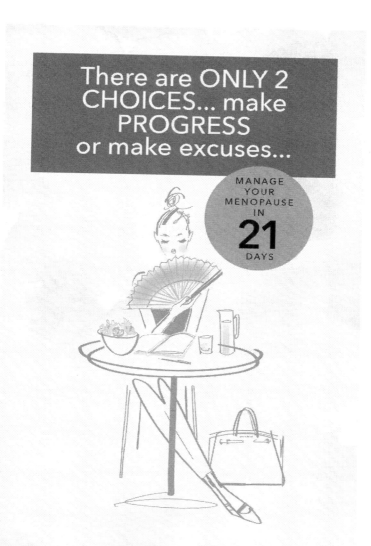

There are ONLY 2 CHOICES... make PROGRESS or make excuses...

MANAGE YOUR MENOPAUSE IN

21

DAYS

INTRODUCTION

Menopause sucks! What other way is there to describe it?

So many of us suffer in silence when it comes to menopause. Most of us haven't got a clue what's happening to our bodies. The person we thought we knew, has vanished! Things that used to work seem to give up overnight and suddenly our waistlines start to expand without control, and we feel bloated and puffy for no reason.

Our hair thins, skin sags and bodies start to ache in places we didn't think could ache. Our brains are like sieves trying to remember the simplest things, our sex drives plummet and finding the energy to get through a day can be tough, especially when one minute you want to cry and the next you want to punch someone in the face!

And the sweating is something else! Who knew we could sweat so much, so often and so ferociously!

As women we know menopause is an inevitable stage of life, but nothing truly prepares us for the impact to our health, minds and bodies. It's been a taboo subject for so long and there are so many myths about treatments and how to manage it, that most of us have no idea where to start, if there is actually anything we can do or is it best just to suffer in silence like our parents did?!

So, if you're struggling with any of the three stages of menopause, this book will really help you understand why you're experiencing the discomfort and changes you're going through and most importantly you'll be given the tools you need to manage your symptoms, along with showing you ways to feel better in just 21 days.

We all need to start somewhere and even if you're feeling at your lowest point right now, know that in less than 21 days you can feel so much better, happier and less bloated with many of your symptoms eased or gone.

My 21 Day Menopause Programme is no magic pill or quick fix fad diet. It's an easy-to-follow programme to help you regain control and start the process of getting you back on track, reduce menopause weight gain, feel hormonally balanced and give you new, healthy habits to positively cope with the menopause journey!

My name is Ailsa, I'm 50 years old and I've been a fitness instructor and all-round wellness fanatic for over 28 years. Over the past 3 years I've been going through my own menopause journey, dealing and coming to terms with the weird and sometimes scary symptoms of menopause.

I train and exercise with women of all ages in health, strength building, weight loss and nutrition, predominantly women in their 40s, 50s and beyond. Empowering them to take back control over their menopause so they feel energised, happy, less bloated and foggy headed.

When I started my menopause journey, I didn't know what I was going through. You don't wake up one morning and think 'The reason I'm feeling this way is because I'm going through menopause!'

Seemingly from nowhere, I was suddenly getting severe acne, which I haven't had since my teens. I was experiencing major discomfort with digesting foods that I've loved eating most of my life. I couldn't understand why I was feeling anxious all the time and low in self-confidence, questioning every decision I made.

Considering I am a relatively fit person, the weight change and bloating came as a surprise! I started getting extreme lethargy, needing to take mid-afternoon naps to keep me going. I struggled with regular severe headaches, my mood was low for no reason (and I'm a bright happy person normally). All that plus the hot flashes at night, major sweats and insomnia between 2am–4am were tough to handle, and to top it off I also experienced a drop in my libido.

Does any of this sound familiar to you?

The menopause journey is a roller coaster, that once you're on, you can't get off. I still have symptoms that turn up unannounced and present a daily challenge. However, through lots of research and working with clients, I've found some really helpful ways to manage the symptoms, get through the tough times and keep a little more balance during the most challenging change a female body has to go through.

Let's face it, the menopause is one thing that ALL women will go through. The average age for a woman to reach menopause is 51, but your genetics, any cancer treatments or other underlying medical conditions can mean you could go through it a lot earlier.

The tricky thing is that no two menopauses are the same. There are so many shades, variations, symptoms and dilemmas to navigate, and in the first instance you don't even realise that it could be related to menopause.

I mean who really feels their age? I know I don't. As crazy as it sounds, I still feel like I'm my early 30's! So... when I reached 47 and all these changes started to happen my first thought wasn't, 'Oh I'm in my late 40s, therefore I must be starting menopause.' No, of course not. No woman wants to think of herself as getting old. I just thought it was stress, my time of the month, eating poorly or maybe going slightly crazy...!

I'd happily take any diagnosis other than the stigma of it being menopause. So, to accept that I was starting to age and that my body was stopping creating hormones that I've depended on most of my life, was no easy feat.

If you're reading this book, you're probably going through a range of symptoms that have started to take their toll on you and you're looking for ways to get a handle on them!

So... a big well done to you!

After all, picking up this book means that you're ready to accept that you might actually be menopausal and that's the first step.

When something like menopause comes along making us feel uncomfortable in our own skin, often very low and unable to cope, it's very difficult to give ourselves permission to take time to stop and really deal with it.

My visit to the doctor was pretty useless too. With no constructive advice, just that I might be depressed or that it's '*that*' time in my life! I wasn't told what I could do, what treatments were available or given any reassurance that it would ease and in the long run I'd be OK.

I'm the kind of person that likes to know the reasons behind why things happen, as that usually gives me a base to understand – or at least try to understand – what the best course of action is to resolve an issue.

I dealt with my menopause symptoms in this way. I wanted to regain some semblance of control and created this programme, that's helped me reduce – and in most instances eradicate – many of my menopause symptoms. And I know it will help you too.

This programme is like a road map for you to follow, so that you can stop hitting dead ends or getting lost on back roads and instead take the fast lane to a stronger, happier, more positive you.

I'm going to be honest – some days will feel harder than others, but if you follow what I recommend for just 21 days, I can show you how to get your body confidence back, stay energised and help you spend a little more time taking care of yourself. You'll then be able to handle all the menopause has to throw at you – and rediscover your lost get up and go!

To get the most out of this book I recommend you read all the way to the end to learn everything you need to know about menopause and what to do on the 21-day programme.

I will give you access to my website that supports the book that will give you workouts, meal plans, a nutrition guide, a daily schedule, journal pages and additional support to ensure you have success.

Plus… at the end of this book in the Appendix are daily motivational messages to help you stay on track and keep a positive mindset.

So, let's not waste any more time, let's get started …

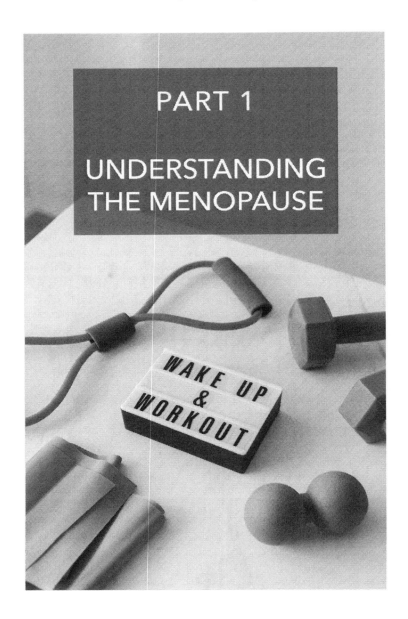

PART 1

UNDERSTANDING
THE MENOPAUSE

CHAPTER 1

THE STAGES OF MENOPAUSE

'Exercise is like life. The harder it is, the stronger you become.'

Let's start with understanding what's happening to us!

A little back to basics, so that we're all on the same page with what menopause is and why we go through it.

No one menopause is the same and every woman over 40 will go through it. Back in the early 1900's our lives were a lot shorter and we didn't live past our 40's. Back then our body's sole purpose was to reproduce.

Fast forward to the 21st century and now we live into our 80s or 90s, nearly double what we used to. As we age, our bodies decline, and as part of that process, women have to live through the depletion of the hormones that have supported their bodies since puberty.

Research into the menopause is still very 'early days' relatively speaking. If you think about it, it wasn't really spoken about by our parents, and many women can't ask their mothers or grandmothers about their menopause as it is still seen as a very personal and private experience.

So, exactly what is happening to our bodies during this time?

Often called the "change of life", menopause marks the end of a woman's ability to reproduce.

When we go through menopause, ovulation stops and our bodies stop producing the reproductive hormones oestrogen and progesterone. As a result, we no longer experience menstrual periods.

There are many symptoms related to the menopause, and they can be different for everyone. In fact, there are as many as forty symptoms that can appear during this phase of life – some of which we would never have imagined to be connected to the menopause.

THESE FORTY SYMPTOMS ARE:

- Hot flashes

- Cold flashes

- Night sweats

- Feeling clammy

· Heart palpitations

· Irritability

· Mood swings

· Trouble sleeping

· Irregular periods

· A low sex drive

· Vaginal dryness

· Fatigue

· Anxiety

· Depression

· Lack of focus

· Poor concentration

· Faulty memory

· Incontinence

· Itchy and crawly skin

· Achy joints and muscles

· Tense muscles

· Sore breasts

· Headaches

· Digestive issues

· Bloating

· A worsening of existing allergies

· Weight gain

· Hair loss or thinning

· More facial hair

· Dizziness

· Vertigo

· A changed body odour

· Electric shock feelings

· Tingling extremities

· Bleeding gums

· Burning on your tongue or the roof of your mouth

· Chronic bad breath

· Osteoporosis

· Weakened fingernails

· Ringing in the ears

With such a huge array of symptoms, menopause can look very different for every woman. You won't experience all of these symptoms, you may only experience a dozen or so, however, to see such a list of what changes can happen to your body – and knowing that you're not in fact 'going crazy'... is an important first step to managing them.

The 3 Stages of Menopause

The term "menopause" can be used to describe the time before, during or just after your last period. We consider there to be three stages of menopause: peri-menopause, menopause and post-menopause.

Peri-Menopause

This is the time when your body is approaching menopause. This generally happens between the ages of 45 and 55. As you approach menopause, your body begins to produce less "female" hormones such as oestrogen and progesterone, leading to a fluctuation in hormone levels. At this time, your menstrual cycle may become longer, shorter or irregular and bleeding can be lighter, heavier or unpredictable. It can also be more painful.

When peri-menopause starts, it is the reduction in oestrogen that has the biggest effect on the body. And when your hormones start to fluctuate so dramatically, major changes to your feelings can occur from out of the blue!

You'll often experience heightened pre-menstrual tension, feelings that are completely irrational, going from happy one minute to crying in a corner the next.

Low confidence, anxiety and stress are also common, and you might have no tolerance of people around you. The emotional rollercoaster can also be made worse by some of the physical menopause symptoms you are experiencing.

The peri-menopause stage lasts for an average of four years. But again, this varies a lot from person to person and the symptoms are a lot more severe at this stage as your body helter-skelters towards full menopause.

My peri-menopause started in a slow, messy way. It wasn't a change in my periods that I noticed at first, although looking back, my cycle had been slightly inconsistent since puberty, so I just assumed it was just another erratic time.

For me it started with the return of teenage acne appearing around my jawline and neck. A problem that I hadn't had for years. This happened alongside feelings of heightened anxiety about doing activities or work that I would usually be confident about performing.

Then the digestive issues of bloating, flatulence, chronic tummy aches and nausea came, and that was a real 'what the hell is happening' moment. I have always loved food and have never been a fussy eater! And to suddenly have severe reactions to food was a very difficult time as I didn't understand why it was happening.

The time that I started to recognise that this could all be linked to peri-menopause was when I started to wake up at around 2am in the morning drenched in sweat. I wasn't just slightly hot, but absolutely drenched - like I was hot from the inside and just couldn't cool down!

I have always leant towards being a cold person temperature wise; I like the heating on, I love a hot water bottle, I like to cosy down under the covers – and now I was throwing off the duvet and having to change my pjs in the middle of the night to ease the sweating.

At that point, I wasn't even familiar with the term "peri-menopause", but funnily enough, it was the hot sweats that made me wonder if my body might be beginning the menopause transition.

I went to the doctor about my symptoms and was told there was no test that could really tell me if I was starting the menopause. I was just given a prescription for my acne and sent on my way.

Many women I know have told similar stories. They started to experience crazy mood swings or low libido or dry itchy skin in all areas of their body, and when they went to check with a doctor about what was going on, they were told there was nothing that could be done.

Most of the time, they were not even guided towards advice on how to manage or handle these very real symptoms and most were given anti-depressants for the low mood.

Menopause

Menopause itself is the stage at which you stop having periods. You're considered to be officially in menopause when you go a full year without one.

However, because our periods can be so irregular during this time, actual menopause can take a long time to reach.

Hot flashes, difficulty sleeping, and vaginal dryness are all very common symptoms at this point whilst our oestrogen is declining.

Post-Menopause

Once you have gone a full twelve months without a menstrual period, you are considered to be in post-menopause. You are in post menopause for the rest of your life.

At this stage, the symptoms you experienced during menopause will slowly begin to ease. However, in post- menopause, it is still common to experience symptoms including:

· hot flashes

· mood swings

· irritability

- insomnia

- vaginal dryness

- incontinence

- mental confusion and difficulty concentrating

- depression, and

- headaches.

You will still go through ups and downs in post-menopause, but with the solutions in this book, you will have the ability to understand and handle what you are going through.

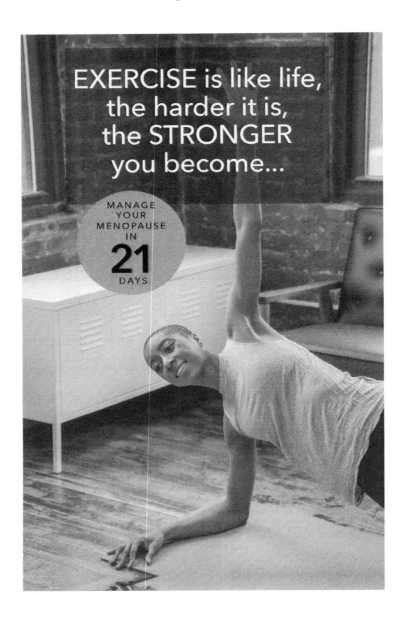

EXERCISE is like life,
the harder it is,
the STRONGER
you become...

MANAGE
YOUR
MENOPAUSE
IN
21
DAYS

CHAPTER TWO

THE EFFECTS OF HORMONE DEPLETION

'During menopause oestrogen drops and cortisol rises. Don't add to the stress by eating less and over exercising. It's all about balance'

While the symptoms of menopause can vary from woman to woman, the vast majority of them are caused by fluctuating levels of hormones in our bodies.

So... we are going to look at hormone depletion in more detail and discover exactly why it wreaks so much havoc on us during our menopausal journey.

What's Happening To Our Bodies?

To understand, let's go back over a little biology to remind ourselves what a monthly cycle is.

During our peak reproductive years oestrogen levels in our bodies fluctuate in a predictable way as we move through our monthly menstrual cycle. Oestrogen levels are predominantly controlled by two specific hormones; a follicle-stimulating hormone known as FSH, and a luteinising hormone, or LH, which is responsible for controlling the menstrual cycle.

The follicle-stimulating hormone, FSH, stimulates the ovaries to produce oestrogen and in turn eggs. Once our oestrogen levels reach a certain point our bodies release the luteinising hormone causing the ovary to release the egg from its follicle, a process we call ovulation.

The follicle then produces progesterone, in addition to oestrogen, preparing the body for pregnancy. If pregnancy doesn't occur, the level of progesterone in the body plummets, menstruation occurs, and the cycle starts all over again.

By the time we reach our late 30s our bodies no longer produce as much progesterone as they used to and the number and quality of follicles is also reduced, leading to less oestrogen.

As we enter our 40s, our cycle generally becomes more unpredictable as oestrogen naturally declines with age. Oestrogen levels can plummet and spike, signalling the body to try and produce more FSH in an attempt to encourage the ovaries to create more oestrogen. This drop and sharp increase of oestrogen is the roller-coaster we go through causing some of our severe peri-menopausal symptoms.

There is a blood test available to measure FSH levels which can be used as a way of determining whether a woman is entering peri-menopause, but this is far from fool proof. Even though a high FSH level can be a sign that peri-menopause has begun, a single FSH reading is an unreliable indicator, because day-to-day hormone levels can fluctuate dramatically, depending on where we are in our cycles, particularly as we get older. Therefore, many doctors don't offer this blood test readily.

What Are The Effects Of Hormone Depletion?

In Chapter 1, I listed out the array of menopause symptoms, but from this list, there are a handful of symptoms women struggle with during "The Change" that seem to be more frequently experienced. Weight gain, hot flashes, fatigue and low libido are four of the most common symptoms most women (not all) go through.

Now let's look at these in a little more detail and uncover exactly what's going on in our bodies when we experience them.

Starting with **Weight Gain**

Weight gain is probably one of the most common side effects of menopause. Putting on weight during menopause is something that can happen very easily – about 30% of women between the ages of 50 and 59 are considered obese.

So, what's the link between our hormones and our weight? Are lower levels of oestrogen to blame for this symptom as well?

The answer is yes, to some degree. Oestrogen plays a number of important roles in the body, including maintaining bone health and regulating cholesterol levels. It can also affect our metabolic rate; that's the body's ability to convert stored calories into working energy.

Reduced levels of oestrogen affects the body's ability to use starches and blood sugar, which increases the levels of fat stored in the body and makes it harder to lose weight.

If you are prone to gaining weight during menopause you are more likely to carry the weight around your tummy and mid-section.

Fat tends to gather around the organs in the abdomen, where it is known as visceral fat. Visceral fat is one symptom of menopause that we need to be particularly careful of, as it has been linked to heart disease, stroke, diabetes and some cancers.

But the weight gain experienced during menopause is not solely caused by lower levels of oestrogen. Many women find that, as they age, they become less active, meaning they burn fewer calories throughout the day.

When we age our bodies have a slower metabolism and each decade, we need less calories per day than we did in the previous decade. When we reach our 50's we need approximately 200 less calories a day than we did in our 40s.

On top of this, there's the fact that lowered oestrogen – along with the natural process of aging – makes us less likely to be physically active. A recent study by the World Health Organisation showed that 1.4 billion adults globally – and a huge one in three in the UK ¬ were not getting enough exercise.

Not surprisingly, our propensity for exercise decreases as we get older. The body's natural aging process also causes us to lose muscle mass, which further decreases our metabolism and makes it even harder to lose weight.

So, keep in mind that as we age, we have to work harder to burn the same amount of calories than we did in the past. That means, in order to stave off weight gain, we need to do a number of things.

We need to eat more consciously, we need to be aware of the food we eat and the portion sizes we consume. We need to move more and we need to lower our stress levels to help our bodies use the energy we store.

The 21 Day Programme focuses on good nutrition and being more active, and offers specific types of exercise, so we get more movement into our daily lives. See part 3 for more information.

Let's talk about **Hot Flushes**

Hot flushes, known scientifically as vasomotor symptoms, are one of the most common symptoms of perimenopause, affecting around 85% of menopausal women.

Hot flushes usually come on suddenly and tend to last between one and five minutes. They can range in severity from a short-lived feeling of warmth to the sensation of being on fire from the inside. Hot flushes can trigger sweating, chills, flushing on the face and upper body, and sometimes even confusion.

Like so many symptoms of menopause, the severity and frequency of hot flushes can vary greatly from person to person, with some women having just a couple a week, and others experiencing more than ten a day and throughout the night.

Though scientists have been studying hot flushes for more than 30 years, they're still not entirely sure how or why they occur. We do know that oestrogen is the main culprit, as oestrogen replacement therapy, or HRT, has been proven to relieve the symptoms of flushes. (We'll discuss this further in Part 2, Chapter 3.)

Let's briefly look at **Fatigue**

Fatigue is another well reported symptom of menopause. Again, the extreme tiredness many women experience during menopause is a result of hormonal fluctuations.

Along with fluctuations in oestrogen and progesterone, our levels of thyroid and adrenal hormones are also all over the place. All four of these hormones are responsible for regulating cellular energy in the body, and when they are unbalanced, you can feel exhausted – seemingly for no reason.

Thankfully, there are a number of ways to manage menopausal fatigue, which we will look at in detail throughout the book.

Low Libido

Another silently suffered symptom is a low libido as well as vaginal atrophy and pain during intercourse.

Many of the women I speak to are suffering with low libidos, vaginal dryness and itchy skin around different parts of their bodies. This subject is rarely discussed openly, but more recently Davina McCall highlighted and brought some much needed attention to it, in her television programme 'Sex, Myths & Menopause', on Channel 4.

Many women struggle with these symptoms in silence. They feel embarrassed, lonely and isolated, thinking they're going through it alone.

Our libidos are important to us. It's our libido that helps keep our emotional connection with our partners; kissing, hugging and sexual intercourse releases oxytocin, which is the love hormone, that makes you feel comforted, connected and sexually aroused.

And while there is no 'normal' when it comes to how often you want or have sex, a low or lost libido can be an additional cause for anxiety and stress during menopause.

When your libido drops or feels like it disappears, you may feel like you don't want to be touched, you have no inclination to have sex and you can feel very disconnected and lonely.

Our sex drives are affected by oestrogen and testosterone. Although it is not widely discussed, testosterone levels drop during menopause. It's testosterone that helps women have a positive sex drive, brain clarity and energy.

The drop in testosterone can be felt more in post-menopause once oestrogen and progesterone are no longer in the body.

The best way to maintain your libido and keep your body functioning as normally as possible, is to keep active and choose a healthier lifestyle.

Exercise and an active lifestyle releases endorphins and increases blood flow to the vagina. This will keep your libido higher, as your mental and physical state will be healthier and in turn your hormones more balanced.

A natural supplement of magnesium can also help stop testosterone attaching to protein cells in the body, so it can roam more freely and be more active in your body.

Alternatively, you can seek help from your doctor who can check your testosterone levels and prescribe a testosterone gel or cream to help balance your levels.

Herbal supplements including zinc, rhodiola and evening primrose oil can also help lift a low libido.

Vaginal dryness and itching is caused by a drop in oestrogen. Oestrogen affects your skin and the amount of blood getting to areas like your vagina, which uses oestrogen to maintain its lubrication and flexibility.

The change in oestrogen levels can cause shrinkage to the vagina over time, in a condition called vaginal atrophy. This shrinkage is what can cause pain during intercourse.

But again, there are ways to manage this.

Firstly, HRT will help reduce the likelihood of vaginal atrophy and relieve dry itchy skin as it boosts oestrogen levels being lost in your body.

If you are unable to take HRT, then exercise can be a big help and taking care of your pelvic floor with strengthening exercises like Kegels and making sure you empty your bladder regularly will encourage blood flow and control.

To ease the symptoms of dryness, shrinkage and itchiness, which can be misdiagnosed as thrush, there are several oestrogen creams, vaginal tablets and oestrogen rings that can be used as a topical application to the area.

Oestrogen creams can help reduce pain during intercourse and relieve itchy sore skin in those delicate areas. These solutions are not the same as HRT and do not have the same associated risks.

They can be used to help maintain a healthy vagina and only affect the area they are in contact with. You will need to talk to a doctor about this to get it prescribed and ask for advice on which one is right for you.

If you are looking for a non-hormonal cream, then you can get vaginal moisturisers via a prefilled applicator, water or oil- based lubricants for use prior to sex. These are not the same as oestrogen gels as they are only useful for enabling sex and won't help relieve the symptoms long term.

4 Hormones that Affect Menopause – which hormone type are you?

There are 4 additional hormones that can also affect your mental and physical wellness during menopause and understanding which hormone you are more predisposed to, will help guide you to your best results.

Type One: The Adrenal Body Type

To identify if you have an issue with your adrenal hormones, you will have a sagging lower belly. The adrenal gland is located on top of the kidneys and produces the hormone cortisol that helps your body manage stressful situations.

When you produce too much cortisol, the body directs the fat to the belly, where it is used as a fuel source for the liver, kidneys and pancreas. If you are prone to high levels of anxiety during menopause you will notice an increase in the stores of adipose tissue fat around the lower belly.

An adrenal body type is generally caused by excess stress, and it can lead to difficulties relaxing or sleeping. The stress of modern life along with high-sugar and processed diets, makes the adrenal body type the most common of the four.

Type Two: The Oestrogen Body Type

If you have been prone to excess weight around your thighs, hips and stomach, it can signify an ovary or oestrogen body type. As we know, the ovaries are responsible for making oestrogen this can create a lining of fat, depositing it around the pelvic and thigh area.

If you have this body type, you are likely to experience significant mood swings, discomfort and irregularities in your menstrual cycle. If you add anxiety into the mix then this body type can transform into the adrenal body type, making the body hold more of its fat stores around the tummy as well as thighs and hips.

Type Three: Liver Body Type

A liver body type is characterised by slim legs and a pot belly that sits high under the ribs. So instead of just lower belly fat you will also have fat above your navel under your ribs. With this body type, the liver is not functioning to its optimal level, leaking fluid into a sack around the middle and causing the belly to protrude.

Some of the symptoms of a liver body type include a slight yellow tinge to the eyes and dark yellow urine, even when you're properly hydrated. You might also experience brain fog during your menstrual period, and deep crevices or a white film on your tongue.

People with liver body types generally have low moods in the morning, pain and tightness in the right side of the body, particularly in the neck and shoulder area. A liver body type can lead you to crave foods such as ice cream, sour cream and cheeses.

Type Four: Thyroid Body Type

Fat evenly distributed around the body is generally a sign of a thyroid body type. The thyroid gland is responsible for controlling every cell in the body and produces hormones that regulate our metabolic processes. If you have symptoms including dry skin and hair, thinning eyebrows, puffy eyes, and cold hands and feet, it could be a symptom of thyroid issues.

Your skin may lose its elasticity and ridges often form on the nails and teeth. An over-active or underactive thyroid can also cause you to feel hopeless or overwhelmed, and thyroid issues are often being misdiagnosed as depression.

Knowing your hormone body type will help you understand your menopause symptoms.

In Part Three, we'll be looking at how to manage nutrition, eating habits, lifestyle changes and movement, to help resolve symptoms associated with your hormone body type.

A Quick Recap!

You now have an understanding of the 3 stages of menopause, the 40 symptoms that can show up on your menopause journey, including 4 of the most common ones, plus you now have an idea of what hormone body type you have that can also have an impact on your menopause.

It's now time to look at ways to help you overcome menopause symptoms and start feeling like your old self again. Remember, the menopause journey is different for everyone, and it's important to consider your own personal lifestyle, health and individual symptoms, to work out which approach is best for you.

In this next section, before we start going through the 21 Day Programme, we will look at HRT (Hormone Replacement Therapy) As well as a more natural route to managing the menopause.

There are still so many inaccurate, scare-mongering stories relating to HRT. So, it's important to know the facts and what options are available, so you can make the right decisions about how to deal with your symptoms.

Both of these avenues will work alongside the programme. If you have thought about HRT, but still feel a little worried or unsure, rest assured, I'll map out the pro's and cons of everything for you to consider. Also, if you prefer to go down the natural route of dealing with your menopause, there are certain foods and natural herbal supplements that can support you.

Most importantly menopause is all about balancing hormones and knowing what you can do will help afford some
control over how you manage yourself going into later life.

Let's look at Hormone Replacement Therapy first.

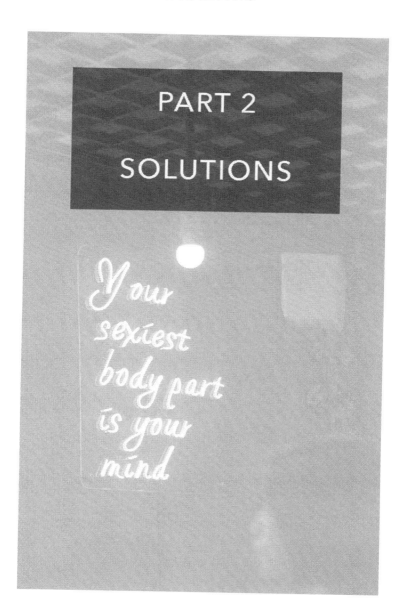

PART 2

SOLUTIONS

Your sexiest body part is your mind

CHAPTER THREE:

THE HRT ROUTE
HORMONE REPLACEMENT
THERAPY

'The question isn't can you, it's will you!'

While it's certainly possible to manage your menopause symptoms without medication, it doesn't mean that approach is for everyone.

Hormone Replacement Therapy, or HRT, is available whether you are in peri-menopause, menopause or post-menopause (as long as you haven't been without oestrogen for 5 years or more).

HRT replaces the hormones that a woman's body no longer produces because of the menopause. The two main hormones used in HRT are oestrogen and progesterone.

Dispelling Myths about HRT and 'The Hyped-Up Risks'

In the 1990s two of the largest studies of HRT users were undertaken, one clinical randomised trial in the USA by Women's Health Initiative (WHI) and one observational questionnaire study in the UK called the Million Women Study (MWS).

The published results of these two studies during 2002 and 2003 raised concerns regarding the safety of HRT. These safety concerns revolved around two main issues:

1) That the extended use of HRT may increase the risk of breast cancer and 2) That the use of HRT may increase the risk of heart disease.

The results of the studies received wide publicity, creating panic amongst some users and new guidance for doctors on prescribing HRT.

However, the women studied in the WHI were North American women in their mid-sixties, often overweight and thus totally unrepresentative of women in the UK for whom HRT might be considered suitable. These would usually be around the age of the menopause, namely 45-55 years.

After the results were published, the UK regulatory authorities issued urgent safety restrictions about HRT, recommending that doctors prescribe the lowest effective dose for symptom relief, to use it only as a second line treatment for the prevention of osteoporosis and advised against its use in asymptomatic postmenopausal women.

Therefore, understandably there still remains widespread confusion and uncertainty amongst both doctors and HRT users because of these original studies.

Findings from Research in 2020

More recent research by the WHI (Women's Health Initiative) was published in 2020, that performed a long-term randomised set of clinical trials and this showed a significant reduction in breast cancer diagnosis and mortality in women using oestrogen only HRT.

Recent evidence from the Collaborative Group on Hormonal Factors demonstrated that there may be a slight increased risk of some types of ovarian cancer associated with HRT use, but this is small and equates to around 1 extra case of ovarian cancer per 1000 HRT users.

The balance of benefit to harm always needs to be assessed, but appears to have shifted favourably for HRT.

This actually means that users of HRT can be reassured provided:

· HRT is taken for the correct reasons, i.e. to alleviate the symptoms of the menopause.

· The dose and duration of HRT use should be made on an individual basis after discussing the risks and benefits.

· No arbitrary limit should be set on duration of using HRT

· Women are assessed by their GP at least once a year

If women start HRT around the time of menopause the risk of ovarian cancer is very small and there appears to be protective benefits for reducing cardiovascular disease and improved bone density.

The Benefits of Taking HRT

Today, HRT is a very viable option for most women in their 40's and 50's struggling to manage their symptoms through diet and lifestyle changes alone.

HRT can balance hormones to reduce or eliminate menopause symptoms like hot flashes, night sweats, mood swings, brain clarity, fatigue, vaginal dryness and low libido.

It improves sleep and skin quality, as oestrogen is an essential for building and retaining skin cells. HRT is also recognised to lower your risk of heart disease, of developing Alzheimer's and dementia as well as lowering your chances of getting osteoporosis and losing bone density.

If you have tried to improve your lifestyle with health changes, but you still feel pulled down, especially mentally by lack of confidence, anxiety, feeling distressed and your normal coping mechanisms are not working then this could be your signal to try HRT and find relief.

Heart disease is one of the most common diseases that women in their 50's suffer from and HRT helps reduce the risk of getting this.

The Risks of Taking HRT

While HRT is nowhere near as dangerous as you may have been led to believe, it is not completely without side effects, and it's important that you are aware of these before deciding whether to go down the HRT route.

The American College of Obstetricians and Gynaecologists has linked HRT to a small but increased risk of breast cancer, deep vein thrombosis, heart attack and stroke. But these are low increases and it is best that you check in with your doctor regularly to evaluate the risks and benefits. Poor lifestyle choices that lead to obesity and diabetes also increase these risks to women's health.

HRT has been controversial since it was first used in the 1960s, but the recent studies have determined that, for women under the age of 60 starting it alongside their menopause, the benefits of HRT far outweigh the risks.

Who can take HRT?

As with anything, one size does not fit all, as each of us experiences menopause in different ways. It's worth exploring HRT as an option so that you understand what is possible for you.

You will be advised not to take HRT if you have a history of breast cancer, ovarian cancer or womb cancer, have a history of blood clots, have untreated high blood pressure or liver disease.

The best time to start HRT will be in the early stages of menopause, but you can take it anytime up to 5 years after your last period whilst your body still recognises the effects of oestrogen.

What's the best way to take HRT ?

Hormone Replacement Therapy is delivered in many ways. HRT can be taken daily, either orally in tablet form or as a gel that can be rubbed on your arm and absorbed. It can also be administered via a skin patch subcutaneously, which can be changed weekly or twice weekly.

Your doctor will advise and prescribe a dosage on how much to use and how to vary it when you need to. Many doctors prescribe gel or patches as there is less risk of clotting and it is absorbed easily through the skin.

Another type of oestrogen that is available is vaginal oestrogen, which can be delivered in a vaginal tablet, cream or ring to help ease itching and dryness to this area of your body.

There is also an option for bio-identical hormone replacements, developed as identical molecules to those produced by the body. These "bio-identical" hormones carry the same benefits and risks as HRT products produced by pharmaceutical companies, but there is absolutely no evidence that the bio- identical hormones are any safer than those used in traditional HRT.

Doctors will advise on dosage levels and it may take a little while to get your dosage correct, but when you do it will help ease your menopause symptoms and allow you to rediscover your old self.

When can I take HRT & for how long?

If you don't start taking HRT when your menopause symptoms start, there is a five year window available to you, if you choose to go on it, post menopause. The time limit exists because as your body goes on without natural oestrogen, it will get used to not having it.

You can take HRT indefinitely – there is no time limit to taking it. When you are post-menopausal you can stay on HRT as long as you feel it benefits your body and mind.

Women wishing to start HRT should carefully discuss the benefits and risks of treatment with their doctor to see what is right for them, taking into account age, medical history, risk factors and personal preferences.

I currently don't take HRT, but I am open to taking it if at any point my symptoms become more severe or if I choose to take it for the advantages it gives my body and mind.

I know that with my family history of osteoporosis and heart disease, HRT would give me the best chance of avoiding the impact of those diseases on my body in later life.

So, if the natural route through menopause doesn't work for you or changes over a period of time, then be flexible and open to trying HRT. The additional hormone support it gives women can make the menopause journey smoother and less stressful.

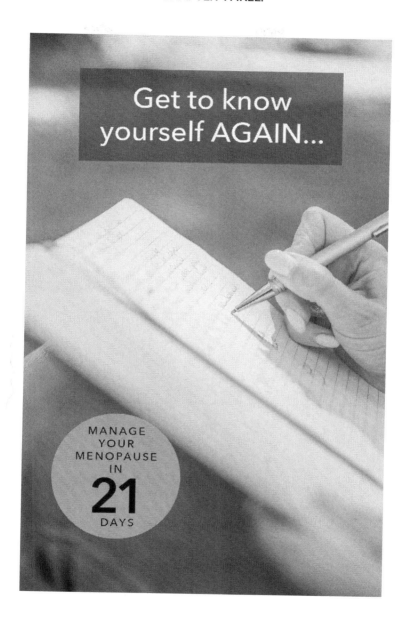

Get to know
yourself AGAIN...

MANAGE
YOUR
MENOPAUSE
IN
21
DAYS

CHAPTER FOUR:

THE NATURAL ROUTE

*'I can't believe I forgot to go to the gym today! That's
7 years in a row now!*

The alternative to choosing HRT is to look at a more natural route through menopause and choose nutrition, herbal supplements and vitamins to support your changing body and mind.

You can add natural oestrogens into your diet and look for specific herbal supplements or vitamins to tackle specific symptoms instead of having the overarching effect of HRT.

In this chapter I am going to outline the ones that can help you through menopause alongside doing the 21 day programme, so you have a balanced approach to all avenues available to you.

Foods That Will Help Balance Hormones

One of the easiest ways to balance your hormones during menopause is to look at what you're eating and use foods to help balance your metabolism and hormones.

To help you with this I want to go through a range of foods called phytoestrogens which naturally support oestrogen in the body. The word 'phyto' meaning 'plant'. These foods exert the same effect as the hormone oestrogen.

Phytoestrogens are much weaker than human oestrogen, so they are not as potent as HRT, which is measured and prescribed. However, the effects of phytoestrogen foods are undeniable.

If we look at the Asian population, who eat a diet heavy in these foods, we can see that their diet supports them in a way that reduces the risk of cervical cancer, heart attack and heart disease, along with the symptoms of menopause.

The Asian population have around 40-60mg of oestrogen a day in their diet, compared to the USA and European diets that have less than 3mg a day!

Foods that have isoflavones, lignans, bio-flavinoids and coumestans are what we need to look for. But you won't see these words on food packaging, so there are few things that you need to look out for.

Isoflavones

Isoflavones are predominantly found in soy-based foods. When it comes to managing the symptoms of menopause, the benefits of soy are never-ending. It decreases hot flashes and migraines, reduces the severity of night sweats and helps regulate your periods, if you still have them.

It's also proven to decrease irritability, mood swings, dry skin and PMS. Soy also makes your hair and nails stronger and helps prevent weight gain by decreasing fat and increasing lean tissue mass.

The benefits of soy are not just limited to the symptoms of menopause. It also reduces your risk of breast cancer, uterine and colon cancer and helps prevent heart attacks by lowering your cholesterol. Along with all that, it also helps reduce the amount of calcium lost by the body, helping prevent bone loss and osteoporosis.

Soy comes in many forms so doesn't need to be boring! You can choose soya beans, called edamame, tofu, soy milk, soy-based meat substitutes, or soy-based dairy substitutes like soy cheese, yoghurt, ice cream and soy protein powders. And if you're looking for a food really high in isoflavones, try fermented soy, known as tempeh.

Lignans

Lignans have powerful anti-cancer properties, particularly among post-menopausal women.

Flaxseeds contain lignans and are a great way to help boost oestrogen levels in the body. Flaxseeds are an excellent source of fibre, and help decrease bad LDL cholesterol, while increasing good HDL cholesterol in the body.

They are also an excellent source of Omega-3 fatty acids, which help reduce chances of heart disease and stroke. They contain plenty of antioxidants and fibre, which improves your digestive health and can help control blood sugar levels.

I add a spoonful of ground flaxseeds to my daily porridge, but you can also mix it into yoghurt, or bake it into breads, add it to salads, the list is endless.

Bioflavonoids

These are another plant-based compound that can really help you manage your symptoms. Bioflavonoids can be found in colourful fruit and vegetables like cherries, blueberries, grapes, cranberries, orange and lemon peel, along with vegetables including peppers and broccoli. You'll also find it in garlic, onions and whole grains.

You can also buy a bioflavin supplement. This daily supplement is recommended at a dose of 1000mg per day.

Coumestans

Coumestans are compounds found in sunflower seeds and bean sprouts and again these foods can add huge benefits like the ones listed above.

Adding these phytoestrogen foods to your daily diet will help to ease your menopause symptoms as part of a balanced nutritious eating plan. You will see in the 21 Day Menopause Programme Meal Plans that there are many of the phytoestrogen foods included to help regulate your digestion, balance out hormone spikes and support your body.

Another Natural Protocol Are Herbal Supplements

Along with phytoestrogen foods, there are a number of herbal supplements that have been successfully used in the management of menopausal symptoms.

Our body's absorption of nutrients and minerals slows and decreases as we age. Supplementing your diet with some healthy vitamins and minerals will help. Plus these will also help ease symptoms, especially if you are not on HRT.

Just remember these alone will not fix you, but as part of a rounded self-care programme they will definitely help

Let's take a look at a few of them:

Evening primrose oil

While there is still only a small body of research regarding the effectiveness of evening primrose oil to treat the effects of menopause, one study showed that, in a group of over 2,000 women who had discontinued HRT, almost 50% of them found evening primrose oil helpful for controlling symptoms such as hot flashes and fatigue. Evening Primrose is a popular supplement for menopausal symptoms.

Black cohosh

This is a flowering plant native to North America and has been used for many years to treat a number of conditions.

Studies show that black cohosh contains compounds that stimulate the body's oestrogen receptors.

It's known to help hot flashes, moodiness, vaginal dryness and excessive sweating. However, as it is not regulated it does have potential side effects. These include jaundice, nausea, vomiting and extreme tiredness. It should not be taken if you are on HRT or hormone therapies.

Red clover

This herbal supplement, just like a number of the phytoestrogen foods discussed, contains isoflavone compounds that act in the same way as oestrogen in the body.

Studies have shown a big increase in oestrogen levels among women who are taking red clover supplements, leading to reduced severity and frequency of hot flashes.

St Johns Wort

Often used to treat depression and alleviate symptoms associated with mood, like nervousness, poor appetite and insomnia. If mood swings and irritability are a big problem for you, this can be a great herbal supplement to try. If you are taking any other medication, check with your doctor first to make sure they are compatible.

Chasteberry

Also known as Vitex Agnus-Castus, is taken for it's hormone-balancing effects. In one study, twenty-three peri-menopausal women were given chasteberry oils, and they reported improved mood and better sleep. In a follow-up study, 33% of participants reported a major improvement in night sweats and hot flushes, with 36% reporting a low to moderate improvement.

There are a number of herbal remedies on the market, but the ones listed above are ones that can specifically support menopause symptoms.

Leading on from these let's look at Vitamins that can also support us.

Vitamins To Help Menopause

Even with the best intentions, a healthy diet doesn't always mean that your body absorbs everything it needs during digestion. Taking additional vitamins can also help manage the symptoms of menopause.

Some of the most useful include:

Vitamin B12: Studies have shown that around 60% of women over 50 have a vitamin B12 deficiency, and this can lead to memory loss, fatigue and insomnia. Taking 1000ug of B12 daily, is a great way to overcome this.

Magnesium: helps the body absorb and retain calcium, which keeps our bones strong and helps fight off osteoporosis. It also helps reduce fatigue, anxiety, headaches and joint paint. Magnesium helps the body to restore energy levels and aids sleep. Aim for a daily dose of 270mg.

Vitamin D: is another great way to keep our bones strong. It's particularly good to take in autumn and winter when we get less sunlight. Symptoms of low vitamin D are bone pain, back pain, muscle weakness, fatigue, tiredness and low mood.

Collagen: During menopause, the drop in oestrogen makes the collagen levels in our bodies plummet. Women lose 30% of their collagen in the first 5 years after going through menopause.

Taking a daily collagen supplement can help keep your skin supple, plump and youthful-looking. There are many products out there but a daily dose from 400 - 8000mcg can help.

Omega-3: can help you sleep better, lowers blood pressure, improves memory, soothes the skin and eases PMS. It also helps boost dopamine levels, reducing the risk of depression and increasing the libido.

An oil blend of omega-3, 6 and 9 may also ease hot flashes and improve bone strength.

Zinc is another great vitamin to take during menopause as it helps maintain collagen and tissue health, and can help reduce vaginal dryness, acne and period pain.

Taking so many vitamins and supplements can be a little overwhelming, so a great solution is to take a good multi-vitamin each day.

There are a number of multi-vitamin supplements available for menopausal women, so talk to your doctor to work out which one is right for you.

The natural route to appease your menopause symptoms is to look at balancing your hormone depletion and what effect that has had on your body.

If you are struggling with the major symptoms of menopause then reviewing changing your nutrition, like including phytoestrogens in your diet, or supporting it with herbal supplements or vitamins to help reduce symptoms are options to consider.

Remember there is no 'magic' pill and there is no quick and easy route to finding what works for you. But the suggestions in this chapter will definitely help you on a natural route to handling your menopause.

We'll be looking at the specifics of our diet in much more detail in Chapter 5.

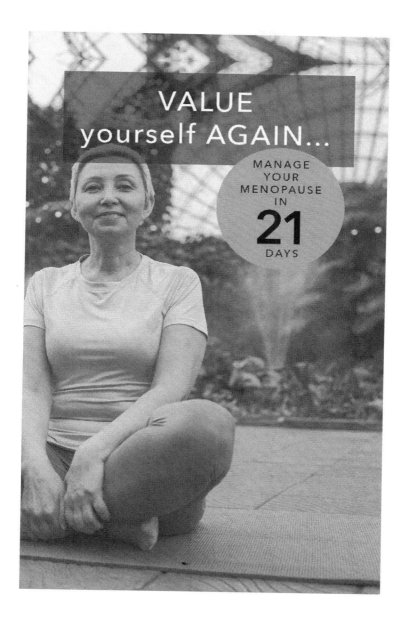

VALUE
yourself AGAIN...

MANAGE
YOUR
MENOPAUSE
IN
21
DAYS

CHAPTER FIVE:

MENOPAUSE AND YOUR DIET

'It took more than a year to gain it. It will take more than a year to lose it'

As food is such an important part of our lives and has a huge effect on our bodies this chapter is aimed at understanding how, what you eat impacts your menopause symptoms.

In this chapter we will look at the links between menopause and diet in far more detail. By the end you will be equipped with a number of helpful tips to understand exactly what the food you eat is doing to your body.

Plus you'll really want to start the meal plans in the 21 Day Programme and get started on making simple changes to your eating habits.

Let's Start with Sugar

One of the most important steps we can take to improve both our menopausal symptoms and overall health is to stop eating sugar or at least reduce it significantly!

As our hormones change during menopause, so does our tolerance to sugar. So, let's just understand what has to happen for our bodies to process it.

According to NHS guidelines, your body doesn't need much sugar to function. People aged 11 years and over only need 30g of sugar per day.

When consumed, the body breaks sugar down into glucose, which is transported via the bloodstream through your body. The pancreas releases the hormone insulin, to help attach to glucose molecules to form glycogen. It is then stored in the body for energy.

If you have a normal daily allowance your body can process what is ingested and produce energy for muscles and organs to use effectively for everyday activities.

However, when we ingest excessive sugar or simple carbohydrates, found in sweets, chocolates, cakes, chips, crisps, fast foods etc. we exceed the 30g daily allowance, this means our poor pancreas needs to keep producing insulin to try and balance blood sugar levels as quickly as possible.

When there is too much sugar in our bodies, the glucose is lain down as glycogen or fat deposits around our tummies, hips and internal organs as adipose tissue.

It's easy to exceed our daily allowance of sugar. An effective way for me to explain this is to look at a favourite drink from a well-known coffee house! Did you know that a grande pumpkin spiced latte has 49g of sugar in it? That's just one drink with well over 19g of a person's daily allowance of sugar.

Add this to anything else you consume in your day and your pancreas and liver will have to work really hard to release insulin to try and keep your blood sugar balanced.

If we keep overloading ourselves with sugar day after day like this, there's a point at which our bodies become less receptive to the effects of insulin and the pancreas struggles to keep up with demand. This can lead to obesity, diabetes and many other health issues. It also leads to constant spikes to your hormones that make you feel sluggish, foggy headed, lacking in energy and low in mood.

If sugar is so bad for us, why do we crave it?

There are several reasons for this:

Did you know that the brain uses more energy than any other organ in the body? And it's main source of fuel is glucose – meaning our mind's ability to function properly is hugely affected by the levels of sugar in our diet.

If you are prone to eating too much sugar, you already know just how addictive it can be. Sugar acts like a drug in the brain's reward centre, stimulating a craving for more, and affecting both our cognitive skills and our self-control.

When we consume sugar, it activates the areas of the brain responsible for creating a reward response. Foods with a high glycaemic index, which means foods assigned a number from 0 to 100, the value of 100 being pure glucose, produce more intense feelings of hunger than low-GI foods. This causes us to feel hungrier and often leads to overeating, especially unhealthy foods and treats.

There's evidence to show that there's an emotional attachment created with foods containing sugar. For example, as a child you may have been given a treat in the form of chocolate or sweets as a way of making you feel better after a fall or as a pick-me-up for feeling bad about something. Our brains associate that treat with easing pain and so it emotionally attaches a feeling to sugary foods and drinks. In later life this can also include alcohol.

As we grow up, we associate the word "treat" with chocolate, sweets, cakes, sugary drinks and alcohol; really anything that has a high sugar and fat content.

Comfort eating is something that we can easily fall into as our brains love and crave sugar, so we eat it. This is how we can get into the habit of reaching for foods that act as a mental and emotional comfort at times when we're tired, have had a bad day, feel lonely, or when we're hurt.

Remember, there is no nutritional value that the body can take from sugar and when we're in menopause, our reaction to sugar is exacerbated, as the drop in oestrogen adds to us feeling fatigued, low and 'hangry'!

When we have an emotional response like this to a hormone depletion, we crave a treat to cheer us up. We grab whatever is closest, usually a biscuit or whatever your "go to" treat is. For those few minutes it's in your mouth it tastes lovely, however, following the sugar high you get an even bigger drop as your hormones, pancreas and liver try to balance out the spike in sugar. You then feel low again and the cycle continues.

When this happens regularly, it creates a habit, leading to weight gain and excessive fatigue.

Menopause symptoms like hot flashes, insomnia, digestive issues, bloating, flatulence, inflamed gut, foggy head, lack of concentration and a lack of energy can also be felt by having excessive sugar in your diet.

Excess sugar consumption is also a major factor in illnesses such as heart disease and type-2 diabetes. Studies have shown that people who consume 17-21% of their daily calories through sugar have a 38% greater chance of dying from heart-related illnesses, than those who consume just 8% of their calories from sugar.

Along with the dangers that a high-sugar diet presents to our heart, it also puts our liver at increased risk of disease. High levels of fructose consumption, the sugar found in sweet beverages like soft drinks and juice, have been linked to fatty liver disease, a condition that now affects about a quarter of the world's population.

As the name suggests, fatty liver results when too many fat cells build up in the liver, greatly increasing the risk of impaired liver function and cancer. Fatty liver can also lead to heart disease, diabetes and kidney disease.

Research has also shown a link between acne and excess sugar consumption. Sugary foods cause our blood sugar and insulin levels to spike, which leads to increased oil production and inflammation, along with a rise in the hormone androgen. All of these have been linked to the development of acne. Which is something I have re-experienced during my menopause.

Something you may not be aware of is that eating too much sugar can also accelerate our skin's aging process. Whilst wrinkles are a natural part of getting older, making bad food choices can cause them to appear earlier and become deeper. This is thanks to advanced glycation end products, or AGEs; the compounds that are formed when sugar reacts with protein in the body. According to scientists, AGEs play a big role in the skin's aging process.

AGEs appear in the body when we eat a diet high in refined carbs and sugar. They wreak havoc on the collagen and elastin in our bodies; the crucial proteins that help the skin remain supple and looking younger.

But it's not just the skin that ages quicker. Scientists believe that excess sugar consumption also causes our cells to age more rapidly. And the more our cells age, the more it hinders our body's ability to regenerate and repair itself in times of injury or stress.

The link between sugar and cellular aging are the body's telomeres, the structures at the end of our chromosomes.

The role of the telomeres is to protect the chromosomes, where our genetic information is stored.

As our bodies age, the telomeres begin to shrink, which can cause cells to degenerate and malfunction. And although this is yet another unavoidable part of getting older, an unhealthy diet can speed up the process.

A 2014 study involving over 5,000 adults showed a definitive link between regularly consuming sugary beverages like soft drinks, sweet teas and premature aging as a result of shortened telomeres. Scientists went as far as to propose that each 500ml serving of sugar-laden soft drink had the effect of an additional 4 1/2 years of aging!

While we often associate sugary foods with that sudden energy hit, the reality is it actually drains our energy.

Sweet foods cause a spike in our blood sugar and insulin levels, which does give us that sudden burst of energy we so often crave. But the energy doesn't last. All too quickly, the energy drops away, causing us to feel even more drained and weary.

This is because when we eat foods that are low in protein, fibre and fat, our blood sugar levels are not maintained. This leads to dramatic swings in our energy levels, which tend to fluctuate wildly during menopause.

It's not just the body that is impacted by too much sugar. Too much sweet food can also wreak havoc on our minds. Research suggests that a diet high in sugar can impact our memory, and even lead to an increased risk of dementia.

Even a small amount of sugar causes inflammation within the brain, which can lead to memory difficulties. But the good news is that this inflammation is not necessarily permanent. When you replace sugary foods with those high in omega-3, such as fish, seafood, nuts and plant oils, it actually improves your working memory.

The reality is that these foods with high sugar and high saturated fats make you feel low, they make you age prematurely, they cause obesity, acne, digestive issues, headaches, hormone spikes, hot sweats (especially when you are in the menopause), insomnia, lack of energy, foggy headedness — the list continues.

During menopause and at any time in your life, the best thing to do is try and ease sugar out of your diet as soon as you can. It will help you revive your energy levels and you will start to feel better and in more control.

We've looked at the effects of sugar to the body, however, this in turn does have an influence on the balance of candida in your gut and your gut health.

Let's look at candida and how to reset it!

When we struggle with sugar cravings that can't seem to be squashed it's not always your hormones affecting you, it could be because your candida is out of control in your gut.

What Is Candida?

Candida albicans is a natural organism (a type of yeast or fungus) that lives in small numbers in even the healthiest of guts. Usually this is balanced by good bacteria that helps to keep this opportunist yeast under control.

If candida is allowed to grow out of control by changes in diet, antibiotics, or stress, it will thrive on the sugars from the food we eat. It then releases toxins which not only have local effects on digestion, causing flatulence, constipation or diarrhoea, but it can have systemic effects too, including headaches, joint pain, foggy head, fatigue, furry tongue, bad breath, urinary tract infections, thrush and those dreaded sugar cravings.

Candida yeast, feasts on simple sugars to survive, so as it gets out of control, it can influence appetite and initiate cravings. Sugar cravings in particular are often an indication that candida overgrowth could be at play, but watch out for cravings for carbohydrates, yeast foods and alcohol too.

So why do we get candida overgrowth in the first place?

Understanding the underlying causes helps to manage the condition:

Diet:

What you eat can be enough to tip the balance of bacteria in your gut. We know that candida and bad bacteria generally thrive on sugar and refined carbs, whilst our good bacteria will thank you for sources of fibre found in prebiotic foods including garlic, leeks, onions and asparagus.

CHAPTER FIVE:

Medications:

Antibiotics are a big problem when it comes to candida, as they affect the good bacteria in our gut which we want to protect us. The contraceptive pill can also affect the natural balance of our hormones which in turn can affect bacteria levels.

Stress Levels:

Chronic stress and poor diet may also influence your chances of developing candida overgrowth. Stress can affect your stomach acid levels and can cause it to become diminished. Sufficient stomach acid is important for regulating the pH and environment of the stomach. To boost your immune system take some echinacea. Echinacea has also traditionally been used as an antifungal.

How do we reset candida levels in our bodies?

Stop feeding candida with sugar and yeast. Cut out common culprits like bread, refined sugar, caffeine, alcohol and Marmite.

Instead, eat natural antifungal and prebiotic foods to help to keep the yeast under control, whilst giving your good bacteria a much-needed boost. Eat lots of fresh vegetables such as garlic, leeks and asparagus plus cooking with coconut oil is a great option.

This may sound obvious, however, it's worth mentioning... chew your food. Most of us simply aren't chewing properly!

The act of chewing breaks down the food we eat and helps to activate the production of some all-important digestive enzymes. Experts recommend chewing your food at least 32 times before swallowing.

These steps will help keep candida under control, plus it's also really important if you suffer from a leaky gut or food intolerances.

Drinking plenty of water, along with eating lots of fresh vegetables will regulate your bowel movements. There are plenty more benefits to drinking water too, which we'll discuss further in Chapter 7.

Pre and probiotic foods support good bacteria, including bananas, miso, yoghurt and tempeh, these can naturally help achieve an optimal balance in your gut.

To help you feel better through menopause and beyond, check in with yourself and recognise that your sugar consumption and /or your candida might be out of control.

Avoid Fad Diets

As women we are bombarded with images on social media, through films and TV advertising, showing us what the "perfect" body and self-image should be. From this, the "diet" industry has become an enormous business. There are countless diets that you can choose to go on, and it all depends on what the current fad is.

Right now Keto is massive, as are fasting diets (which many people think is starving yourself!) which by the way, they are not.

In the past, the Atkins diet, shake diets, raw food diet, paleo diet, the Cabbage Soup Diet and the Beverley Hills Diet were all supposed to give amazing results and we were coaxed into trying them.

We are shown images of before and after shots of women who have achieved amazing results in a short space of time from a supposed 'magic pill', or 'get slim quick' diet. It's aspirational and what we all want to achieve, because isn't it right that "happiness" is found in being slim!!! (I am saying this with tongue-in-cheek sarcasm!)

The reality is that 99% of diets don't work in the long term. If you don't resolve your deep-seated eating issues and what you associate with emotional comfort, then you will always revert back to your original weight as soon as you drop the diet.

Sometimes, because your body thinks you've been starving it, you find that you put on more weight than you did the first time around.

This is also exacerbated when a diet finishes by reverting back to eating, highly processed, high-fat, high salt and sugary foods, that are easily and cheaply available.

When that happens, our brain doesn't just say "I want more of this", it goes into a crazy mode and we overeat and put on weight.

During menopause, with hormone fluctuations and your body being older, you will find that fad dieting will not only mean you put on weight, but you'll also have resulting menopause symptoms that come with the stress of radically changing your diet.

Our brains love to believe that there is a quick fix to our problems. But in truth anything that works for us and stays with us long term includes creating a new habit, and sticking with it until it becomes a new normal.

Stress Eating

As we know, both the hormonal and lifestyle changes of menopause can make us particularly susceptible to depression and frequent low moods. While this is challenging enough in itself, we have also discussed the link between stress, depression and weight gain, particularly among middle-aged women.

The link between our mental state and our weight is largely to do with our eating habits, particularly stress eating which happens as a response to either external stressors, or negative emotions.

This not only leads to plenty of unwanted pounds, but it also makes our mood fluctuations worse – in turn leading us to make poor food choices. It's that same vicious cycle we discussed regarding sugar cravings.

Interestingly, acute stress, such as a near accident while driving, can lead to a decreased appetite, while chronic stress such as financial pressure, family difficulties, or the lifestyle changes brought about by menopause often increases our appetite and our desire for energy-dense foods like biscuits, crisps, butter and cheese.

The mood fluctuations and chronic stress we experience during menopause make us far more likely to engage in stress eating than we did when we were younger.

Recognising that we are stress eating is an important first step in managing it, and reducing the weight gain it can bring about. But what else can we do to help us get on top of this potentially dangerous practice?

Firstly, check in with yourself. Understanding exactly what triggers your stress eating is a powerful way to overcome it. Next time you catch yourself heading for the fridge, take a moment to check in. Are you actually hungry, or are you eating in the hope that it will make you feel better?

If it's the latter, take some time to identify exactly what it is you're feeling. Are you experiencing a low mood or mood swing? Has something specifically stressed you out? Maybe you're feeling bored and listless?

Identifying your triggers and taking the time to name your emotions is an important way to keep stress eating in check. Write them down so that when they happen again you have a better chance of putting a strategy in place to help avoid going down the wrong path of grabbing whatever is at hand to munch on.

Secondly, get rid of temptations. Having chocolate in the fridge, or a jar of biscuits sitting on the counter can make it all too easy for us to eat when we're not hungry.

Research has shown that when we can see calorie-dense food such as sugary treats and chocolate, it stimulates the striatum, the part of the brain responsible for controlling our impulses. This makes it that much harder to resist those treats and can trigger your cravings and overeating.

Do yourself a favour and keep unhealthy, tempting foods out of sight – or better yet, out of your fridge and pantry entirely.

Thirdly, maintain a healthy eating routine. We are more likely to overeat when our eating habits don't follow a schedule. When we eat our meals at random times each day, it disrupts our body's normal process of digestion and can lead to spikes in blood sugar and cholesterol.

When you skip meals, it also means you're much more likely to overeat at the next meal and are more likely to grab unhealthy snacks to stave off the hunger that strikes in between.

Scientists believe that *when* we eat is almost as important as *what* we eat, and this is for a number of good reasons. Eating your meals at the same time each day increases our metabolic rate, helping us burn those calories faster.

Having a meal schedule also helps us make mealtimes a priority; a time in which we choose to nourish our bodies with the right food, instead of making erratic and impulsive food choices and resorting to stress eating.

Fourthly, don't deprive yourself. When we notice ourselves gaining weight, our impulse is often to try and reduce the number of calories we are consuming. But depriving yourself of food when you're hungry and forcing yourself to count calories is a sure-fire way to increase your stress levels. And when that happens, we often find ourselves completely falling off the wagon and bingeing – leading us to feel stressed out all over again.

As we discussed earlier in the chapter, constant dieting is not only an ineffective way to achieve lasting weight loss, it can also increase your stress levels and be harmful for your mental health.

Menopause is no time to be depriving yourself of the things you love, it's a time to take care of your body and feed it with foods that will nourish you and make you feel good.

Instead of counting calories, stock your fridge and pantry with filling and nutritious foods such as avocados, beans, nuts and seeds.

Another thing you can do is go back to making home-cooked meals. Studies have shown that when we regularly digest home-cooked meals, we are increasing our intake of fresh fruits and vegetables, which reduces the severity of menopause symptoms. (We'll be discussing this further in Chapter 7.)

Furthermore, research shows that people who digest home- cooked meals five times a week are 28% less likely to be overweight than those who eat at home just three times a week. When you eat at home, you have full control over the ingredients you are putting into your food – and subsequently your body – so you know exactly how much salt, sugar and fats you are consuming.

So, there you have it, lots of ways that food, nutrition and diet can affect you during the menopause and beyond.

You may be feeling a little overwhelmed by everything I've said but in the next section I will take you through how to Manage your Menopause in 21 days, how to take back control and start yourself on the road to creating new habits, that will support you moving forward with your menopause journey.

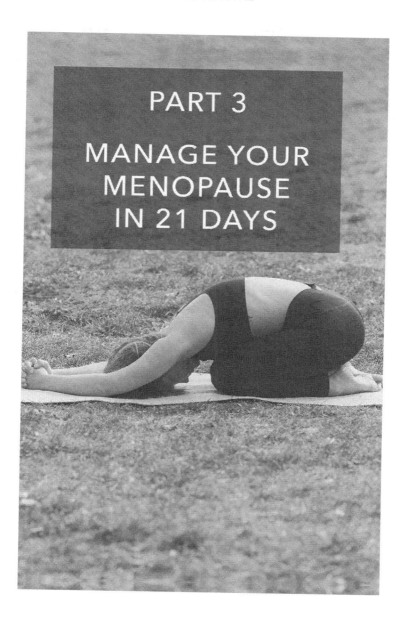

PART 3

MANAGE YOUR
MENOPAUSE
IN 21 DAYS

CHAPTER SIX:

WHAT TO EXPECT ON THE 21 DAY PROGRAMME

'Your body can do anything. It's your mind that needs convincing'

In this section of the book, I will introduce you to the Manage your Menopause 21 Days Programme in detail, so you can craft your own 21-day plan.

While the programme obviously works best if you follow it as closely as possible, life can happen. So pre-plan forward as much as you can and implement the easy- to-follow protocols to help you find the balance you're looking for.

In order to succeed at any programme you need to prepare yourself for success, so let's get started.

Steps To Success

STEP 1 ...Get to Know Yourself Through Journaling

When you start the 21 Day programme it will involve changing some of your daily habits. This is never easy, but one of the best ways to help is to start a journal.

If the thought of this scares you, don't worry, you're not alone! I've never been a diary person, but these days there's lots of different ways to journal, so that you can make it your own.

You can use the 'notes' app on your phone. You can chat into your phone's dictation app. You can choose a lovely notebook with an inspirational front page that makes you want to jot down your thoughts and day's activities. Or you can use the Journal pages that I've created for you, that you can find on my website www.50shadesofmenopause.co.uk.

You can print out the pages with helpful pointers to guide you to making notes on how you're feeling, what you're eating, what exercise you manage to do, how your menopause symptoms are on a daily basis and what self-care activities you're doing to calm your mind and feed your soul.

Whichever you choose, make sure it's a method you know you can sustain for at least a month.

Journaling how I'm feeling, noting any stress I'm going through, symptoms that spring up as a daily challenge, planning forward and off-loading rubbish stuck on repeat in my brain, has been invaluable on my menopause journey.

It's also been a way for me to get to know myself and who I am as a 50-year- old woman.

Sadly, most of us start journaling in times of crisis. Maybe it's at a midlife crossroads, a relationship break-up, losing a job, losing a loved one or dealing with menopause.

I started journaling in the early stages of my menopause having never journaled before. I tend to do mine in the early mornings when it's calm and the family are still in bed. I write down the things that I'm going through, where my head space is, what's bothering me, what symptoms are affecting me and monitor when things are happening in my cycle.

One of my symptoms has been extreme anxiety. I used to constantly worry about running out of time to do everything I needed to do in my day and became obsessively nervous. It would overwhelm me to the point of stopping me in my tracks.

I used my journaling to help me co-ordinate my workloads, family activities and commitments. I also started to write down how I felt when I woke up and how my previous day had been, how I'd slept and what I was doing. As I went through it, I could see patterns starting to emerge.

For example, when I ate my beloved chocolate in an evening watching TV, I would find the next day that I felt tired, headachy, moody and lacklustre. I'd have no energy, tummy cramps, bloating and hot flashes would creep up on me. But when I didn't eat it, I could feel my head space was clearer,

I didn't have an irrational mood swing plus my digestive issues went away.

Journaling my day, times of the month, eating patterns, exercise and stress levels became something that helped me get through some pretty awful times. It made a little more sense of the irrational out-of-the-blue episodes that I was going through and I have also learnt a lot about myself and my habits along the way.

I've made journaling a crucial part of the 21 Day Programme so as you go through it you can get to know yourself better. I have outlined exactly what you need to write down for each of the 21 days, so you can get into the swing of it easily and then start making it your own.

So, on Day 1 you will write out everything you are experiencing right now. From symptoms that you recognise as menopausal, to ones you don't see as related, but are very apparent.

These might include massive mood swings, like feeling okay one day to feeling upset and crying the next. It might be a loss of confidence, anger, frustration, anxiety or not wanting to see anyone.

Also think about what makes you feel good, what makes you feel bad and what your triggers are when it comes to stress, food, work, and family.

What do you do for self-care?

What do you do to self-sabotage your good intentions?

What are your current habits – both good and bad?

We all develop habits through our lives that we think support us, but one of the truths I have learnt over the past three years, is that what works for you in your 20s and 30s, doesn't work for you when you are going through your menopause.

When was the last time you took a look at yourself and your habits? Probably never.

How can you feel happy and healthy if you don't know what makes you tick, and what fills you with joy?

What things did you used to do that made you happy, that for some reason have been put on hold?

Are there things you used to do that are no longer in your life, but you'd like to restart?

This is the time when you really need to take a step back and look at the bigger picture, because all your normal support mechanisms, from food, to activity, to sleep get affected and you don't know how to start helping yourself because everything just feels wrong.

Journaling can be very cathartic. You'll write down everything important to you that you may have suppressed due to circumstances, feeling less than yourself, or just having had to shape yourself to others' wishes.

It can be a challenging exercise, as it can dig up feelings you may not have been aware of; feelings you might rather keep hidden. But don't judge or censor yourself - just get everything down on paper as your truth and you can deal with it from there.

This is your starting point. There's no need to find solutions to any of it yet, and there's certainly no need to feel overwhelmed. All we want to do here is take stock of where we are right now.

Then each day you need to write down how you feel when you wake up, how you slept, what you did before you went to bed, what events occurred that may have made you wakeful, if you had any hot flashes or insomnia and so on.

Plus mapping out what you've eaten, what activities you've done, any self-care you do, and what time you go to bed.

During the programme, you're going to get to know yourself better and see what you need to do to help manage your menopause symptoms as calmly and considerately as possible.

These symptoms are not going to go away by themselves and will be with you for a long time. You might as well get to know what your triggers are and what gives you joy and happiness so you can focus on those things.

At the end of the day, it's about making better life choices for you and creating some very positive changes that will set you up for success for the rest of your life.

STEP 2 ...A Positive Mindset

Mindset and being positive before you start anything new, is critical to success. If you have a positive "Can Do" attitude it will help you on days that feel tougher than others. At the start of any journey, there will always be roadblocks, especially with anything to do with change to your old routine. If you look hard enough, you'll always find a reason not to do something that feels difficult.

When we're faced with something new and difficult, our brains go into protection mode, and that's why diets, or any kind of change of course in life is so tricky to navigate, because we have a default system that kicks in and tries to talk us out of making the harder choice.

The only way around it is to put your new goals in clear sight, start the day with a positive "I can do this" attitude and know that if things get tough you have measures in place to stop you going backwards.

This is where your journal can be a great help. When you've got everything written down in front of you, you can look at your current physical and mental issues and know that the only way out is to keep going.

Remind yourself that tomorrow is a new day, and that with every small step forward, you will be helping yourself get to a better place both mentally and physically.

Set yourself some short-term goals that will stretch you, but that still feel achievable. Find something that will inspire you. Is there a holiday that you want to go on?

Do you want more energy to play with the grandchildren?

Do you want to stop joint pain and go for some long treks with your partner?

What's your thing?

We all need a "why". If you don't have that to help you, it will be harder to achieve your goal.

A visual stimulant is a great way to keep you on track. Write out your goals and put them somewhere you will see them every day or set your phone's background to the place you want to travel to on holiday.

You need to get your family and friends on board to help support and encourage you. We all need a "you can do this" and "you've got this" from others around us, inspiring us to push forward and achieve.

The feeling you get when you achieve your goal is incredible, and the only one that can get you there is YOU.

So, create a goal, get family support and look at your symptoms. Do you really want to stay feeling the way you do? If the answer is NO, then you are ready to get started...

STEP 3 ...Prepare for Withdrawals

As I've said, you're going to make changes to help overcome the symptoms of menopause and one of the elements that needs to be reduced is caffeine.

Many of us depend on a nice cup of tea or coffee to start the day, but caffeine is a stimulant, which spikes our hormones

— and not in a good way. It also dehydrates the body and can cause you to feel groggy and fuzzy headed after the initial high. This is because all the cells in our body, including the brain, need water to keep working optimally.

Rather than completely cutting out caffeine all at once, you can choose in the first instance to lower the quantity of caffeine, say to one cup of coffee per day. You could also switch to decaffeinated options.

You will also be reducing sugar out of our diet. But while cutting down on sugar and caffeine will make you feel great in the long-run, there's no denying that it can be really challenging in the beginning.

When you lower the amount of caffeine and sugar in your diet you will have withdrawal headaches and you can feel emotional and low in mood as your body detoxifies, so be prepared for this. It can last between 24 to 72 hours but once you're through it, you'll feel so much better.

As we cut sugar out of our diets, we are also likely to experience sugar cravings that can tempt us back to our old bad habits. But if you want to make lasting changes, it's crucial not to give in to cravings.

When they do strike — and they will — move and get active, do a workout, go for a walk or drink water. Cravings only last four minutes, and distraction and action are the key to overcoming them.

You can also try cleaning your teeth as nothing tastes great with toothpaste or when your mouth feels clean! And if you have to have a snack then why not go for chopped sticks of carrots or cucumber? They are crunchy and sweet and can help ease the craving.

It's a case of mind over matter at times like this – but I know you can do it! And remember they won't last for long.

STEP 4 ...Prepare to Move

As we get older, most of us become more inactive. This isn't just to do with aging, it is to do with energy levels feeling lower, especially during the menopause when we lose vital hormones that energise us and make us feel good.

But energy and activity, actually creates energy and action! And if you're not active now you will be for the next 21 days! During the programme, you will be adding in daily walks and exercises to help balance your hormones and start to get your body moving.

The benefits of exercise are endless

Firstly, when we get active, our bodies release endorphins, which help us feel good. These hormones counter the cortisol which makes us feel anxious, fearful and lacking in confidence.

When we exercise, dopamine and serotonin are also boosted and these combine to help us feel brighter and more capable of handling our symptoms, our families and normal daily challenges better. It also helps with sleep.

Our mental health is so important. Fresh air, socialising and moving all link together to help lift our mental health and well-being.

Exercising is also a great way to ease achy joints. When our bodies ache, all we want to do is lie on the couch, but the truth is, this is probably the last thing that we should be doing. Our bodies are created to move and in today's modern world, where we spend so much time on social media, watching TV, or working at a computer, we move less and less.

This causes joints to stiffen, our muscles become weaker; they shorten because they're not being stretched and used. Our muscles feed our bones and joints. By using them and strengthening them with a range of exercises, including body weight exercises, we'll get the synovial fluid working, helping to reduce stiffness, aches and pains.

In the next chapter we'll be looking at how to choose the right exercises for you, and how to make movement an integral part of your day-to-day life.

STEP 5 ...Prepare to Feel Days of Doubt

Making lasting change is hard. All too often, our old habits try to return and sabotage our journey.

When we start anything new, we have an excitement and zest for taking on board what's needed and feel motivated to give it our all.

Anything new can feel daunting, but because it's new we give it a go! It's that excitement and motivation for change that drives us to step out of our comfort zones.

We believe that motivation will be enough to sustain us and stop us from going off track. Unfortunately, however, this isn't the case. Your body and mind have developed coping mechanisms over the years and breaking out of long-held habits can be tough – even when you know they're not good for you!

Our brain is extremely clever. It relates our emotions to things that bring us comfort and pleasure. Although we know that too much chocolate, crisps, fatty foods and take-aways are not the best things for our bodies. Our brains will remind us in a low moment that, that's what we need to make us smile!

The fact that there are no nutritional benefits for your body never enters your brain. All you feel is emotional craving. You just need what you're used to having.

Breaking these habits and patterns are the hardest. But this is the time for you to be strong and resist the cravings and NOT go back to your old ways!

So, being prepared and realistic is really important. Under-stand that there will be a day along the journey, when you will have an emotional blip, or it feels harder than others to keep yourself on track.

But know that you're not alone and this is completely nor-mal and there's no need to create a whole load of guilt around it. If you can get support from your family to en-courage you to help you stay on track, you'll have more success of pushing through.

When we do the programme together it's the group cama-raderie that helps the women on the programme! Every step of the way there is support and encouragement from women who know what you're going through – women who can help you when you feel your willpower starting to waver.

You need to make sure, especially in those first seven days, that whatever happens you are ready to use all the options I will give you to push through so you can start seeing the benefits of the programme.

After seven days it will be easier to keep going as you will be well on your way to learning to make those new habits and routines a normal way of life. You will also feel so much better within those first 7 days that it becomes easier to keep going.

I get asked, "What happens if I do stumble and fall back into my old habits?"

Well, my answer is always that it's not the end of the world; pick yourself up and commit to starting fresh again the next day.

If you need an extra boost, or are having a moment of struggle staying on track, then flick to the Appendix where you'll find daily messages that'll give you the boost and encouragement you need.

STEP 6 ...Measurements, Photos and the Fitness Test

When starting the programme, one of the first things you will do will be to take photos of yourself in your sports bra and leggings or favourite underwear. Something that you know you feel comfortable in and can wear each time you do a check-in with yourself.

These photos are not for self-criticism but are a reference point for you to know where you're starting from. You may think you have put on menopause weight around your middle for example and can see how your weight gain is different from before.

Or you might actually realise it's not as bad as you thought. It's much better to see changes through a camera, as scales can lie quite easily depending on the time of day, what you have eaten or drunk, and whether it is your time of the month!

Taking measurements is also important as they will give you a guide as to where you are with your body shape and the way you feel. These measurements, along with the photos, will be kept in your journal and will only be referred back to at the end of the 21 days.

There is a fitness test that I ask you to do either before Day 1 or on your first day. This is nothing to worry about. It's just a way for you to see where you are physically at the starting point of this journey.

It's all low impact movement and there are demonstrations and alternative exercises so you are able to workout to your current fitness level.

This starting point is one for you to progress from. Go to the website www.50shadesofmenopause.co.uk to see the fitness test. At the end of 21 days, test yourself again to gauge your improvement.

Some of the ladies who have done this programme with me had not exercised since they were in their 20s, and by the end were so surprised and pleased with their progress and energy levels. Exercise has now become something that they love doing and choose to do to stay healthy and strong.

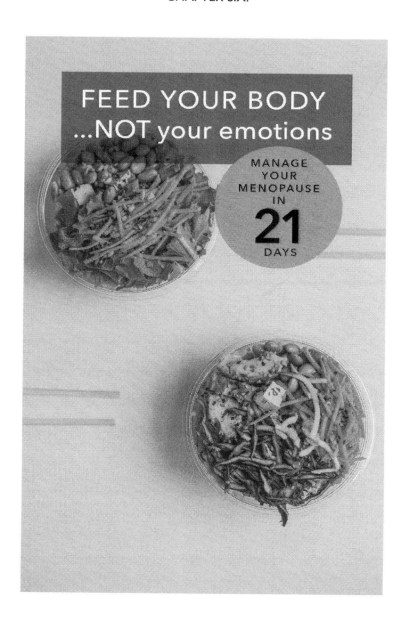

FEED YOUR BODY
...NOT your emotions

MANAGE
YOUR
MENOPAUSE
IN
21
DAYS

CHAPTER SEVEN:

THE FIVE ELEMENTS OF THE 21 DAY PROGRAMME

'Your body hears everything your mind says.' -Naomi Judd

The 'Manage Your Menopause' in 21 Days is made up of five elements. If you manage these five elements on a daily basis as guided, you will see many of your menopause symptoms lessen, your weight gain will stop, and you will feel better mentally and physically.

Consistency and discipline are key to obtaining life-changing results. Once you have learnt these new habits and add them to your daily routine, you will really see amazing changes to your life.

It's an exciting prospect to know that these five elements will help you get your hormones and mood balance back.

Plus give you a clear guide to help you feel stronger, more energised, reduce menopause symptoms and help carry you through your menopause journey and beyond in a more positive way.

The five main elements of the programme are:

Water – Exercise – Nutrition – Sleep and Self-care

Let's take a look at each of them in detail as you will include these in your daily schedule over the 21 days. Knowing the benefits and the "why" for adding these to your day makes them easier to stick to.

1. Water

This sounds so obvious, but it is often underestimated and rarely recognised. Did you know that the cells in our bodies are made up of 70% water? Water is vital for so many functions in our bodies and we rarely drink what we need to maintain equilibrium.

Water helps flush out toxins from the body, it feeds our cells with the energy they need to function, it transports blood, it creates the energy to move and clears the brain, so you feel less lethargic. It also helps your organs function efficiently.

When our bodies are dehydrated, it increases the risk of obesity. Research has shown that when our bodies are larger, they require more water and unless we up our intake, it can create a vicious cycle of weight gain.

Dehydration has also been linked to mood swings, difficulty concentrating and low energy levels – all of which are typical symptoms of menopause – and all of which can lead to stress eating.

All too often, when we experience what we think is hunger, we are actually, more often than not, thirsty. Drinking enough fluids helps you feel fuller and can actually increase your metabolic rate, thereby boosting the number of calories you burn on a day-to-day basis.

When, you drink water is also important. When we wake up in the morning we've been dehydrated for a long period of time. We can wake feeling groggy and lethargic, and during menopause night sweats and hot flashes are very common and will also dehydrate the body.

So as a new daily habit, a great way to start your day will be to drink a lovely large glass of water. You can have it cold, warm with lemon, room temperature, however you like – but try and make a plan to drink a glass of water before drinking anything else in your day.

Also, if you drink a glass of water half an hour before your meal it can help stop you from overeating. In fact, a 2010 study showed that dieters who drank half a litre of water before their meals lost 44% more weight over a three-month period than those who didn't.

Try and drink around eight glasses a day to help maintain balance in your body and mind and don't underestimate just how good water can make you feel.

CHAPTER SEVEN:

2. Exercise

Being told to exercise or work out can feel overwhelming for some women, especially if it's not something you've done for a while or haven't made part of your lifestyle. But exercise should be seen as your friend.

Our bodies are meant to move and as we get older the importance of movement and staying active is even more significant. The saying "If you don't use it, you lose it!" really does apply to us as we age.

When it comes to exercising, it's all about creating new habits, and making it a part of your routine.

So, what can you do to give yourself the best chance of success?

Firstly, speak to your doctor before beginning any new exercise programme. Make sure you are choosing activities that are suitable for your body.

Also choose activities that you enjoy. You're far more likely to give up on a programme if exercise feels like a chore.

If you're not sure what to choose, take a moment to consider whether there are any activities you've always wanted to try. As we talked about in the previous chapter, menopause is the perfect time to try something you have always wanted to do.

Consider the activities you used to love as a child. Maybe you adored ballet dancing, playing netball, badminton, hula hooping or swimming?

Sure, your body may not behave like it used to, but that doesn't mean you can't still enjoy the activities you once loved. Find an adult dance class or see if there are any social sports teams you could join.

Joining a class or a team activity helps to hold you account-able, so too can partnering up with a friend. Finding some-one to exercise with will not only mean you have someone to answer to if you decide not to show up, it also makes exercise a lot more fun!

For the 21 days there are a variety of exercise workouts for you to do on the website. Start with these, but don't be afraid to add in something that you love doing and make it your own special thing.

Finally, pick a start date. Write it in your calendar or put it into your phone. Setting time aside for exercise ensures it doesn't get forgotten in the chaos of day-to-day life, and it's another great way to hold yourself accountable.

Variety is key!

When it comes to exercise, like so many other things in life, variety is key. Most women who start my programme are either non-exercisers or they just run or just walk. There is little variation in their exercise routines.

When we do just one activity our bodies start to get used to it. We adjust quickly and there can be repetitive strain on joints or muscles because there is no variety in the move-ment.

I recommend finding a way to balance this with a range of exercises to develop strength, flexibility, cardio health, balance and core strength. This way your body benefits from not being over-exercised in one area and can keep its full range of movement.

I teach Pilates, Body Conditioning, Legs Bums and Tums, Activation Band and I love to do deep stretch and calming so that your body and mind get the most from a full range of movement.

For the programme I have created a range of workouts for you to do on a daily basis for the 21 Days. The exercises are for all fitness levels, so even if you haven't worked out for a while you can start at a level that suits you. Go to www.50shadesofmenopause.co.uk.

Trying these exercises which mix strength building, toning, improving your body's cardio and stretching will really help you start to feel stronger, build your confidence and get to know what your body is capable of.

We're rarely told of the benefits of exercise – only that we should do it!

So here are the reasons why we should exercise & move:

As we age, our bodies naturally lose more than just our hormones. When we go into peri-menopause we lose muscle tone and are more prone to osteoporosis, the weakening of our bones which makes us more susceptible to injury.

Strength building exercises using body weight or hand weights helps maintain muscle tone and feeds into our skeletons, strengthening our bones and balances the effects of those depleting hormones.

Exercise is important when it comes to avoiding weight gain. During menopause, we gain weight, particularly around the abdomen. Maintaining a healthy weight with exercise and movement helps stave off diseases such as cancer, heart disease and type-2 diabetes.

Regular exercise, particularly during our later years keeps our joints and muscles strong, helps our bowels function the way they should and can help relieve depression and anxiety.

As we age, we need to adjust our exercise habits choosing the right kinds of exercise during our menopause and post-menopausal years, to help us feel strong, maintain flexibility, balance and help our metabolisms stay energised.

During the 21 Day Programme, you are guided every step of the way. There is variety so that we use all our muscles, tone, improve our cardio and strengthen through our core. The workouts can also support any activity you currently do.

So, what kind of exercises are best?

Strength Training

Strength building for women is essential. I'm not talking about building muscles so you are muscley and look like you could enter a body building competition! Unless that's the way you want to go!! No, what I mean is that when we exercise using our own body weight or light hand weights or cans (whatever you have to add a little resistance to your movement!) we help to strengthen our muscles, increase our metabolism, burn fat and strengthen our skeletons.

Using resistance is one of the best things women going through menopause can do to help retain their youth, retain skin tone, balance, core strength and overall mental health.

Using resistance increases the deposition of calcium to the loaded bones which increases their density and subsequently reduces the risk of osteoporosis.

Resistance training also brings about dramatic adaptations to the muscular system in the body and these improvements can improve self-esteem and confidence. As it builds lean tissue in the body it also increases the metabolic rate and this increase in metabolic rate helps to lower body fat.

That's why the majority of the exercises in the 21 Day Programme focus on strength training and targets different areas of the body.

If you don't do so already, be sure to incorporate some resistance strength training into your exercise routine. This might mean using weight machines at the gym, or attending a regular yoga or Pilates class, or simply using a lightweight set of dumbbells (1-2kgs) at home.

Cans of food weigh 350g – 400g and will work just fine if you don't have access to proper weights.

The exercises I guide you through will help you see improvements with your posture and body strength. The aim is to do strength training exercises a minimum of two to three times a week.

Low-Impact Cardio

Low-impact aerobic exercises are great for keeping our heart and lungs strong and healthy. One of the best examples of this type of exercise is walking, as it's something you can do anywhere at any time, and at your own pace.

A walk is simple and easy to add into your day, is great for your mind and is one of the exercises I ask you to do each day whilst on the programme.

Walking is a weight-bearing exercise, which has a huge range of health benefits. Not only does regular walking help with weight loss, it also increases our heart and lung fitness and reduces the risks of heart disease and stroke. It can help manage conditions like high blood pressure, high cholesterol and diabetes. It's a great way to counter muscle stiffness, strengthen your bones and improve your balance and endurance.

Walking for just 30 minutes a day is enough to reap all these benefits. If you find it difficult to walk for 30 minutes at once, start smaller. Aim for three 10-minute sessions per day, or whatever your body can manage. After all, even the smallest amount of exercise is better than nothing!

You may find it easier to get into the habit of taking a daily walk by aiming to do it at the same time each day. I'm a morning walker. I get up early to make sure that I can get out and walk before the family rises and I get quality "Me" time to think, clear my head of stress, energise myself for what the day has to offer, and I know that even if I have a day of sitting at a computer, my body has had a chance to move.

Setting your alarm half an hour earlier and getting out for a walk before work can be a great start to the day. But if the sound of that fills you with horror, no problem! Simply find a time that works for you. You could walk in your lunch break, or after finishing work for the day.

As your fitness improves over the 21 days, you will likely notice yourself being able to cover more and more distance in the same amount of time.

You can also increase the intensity of your walks by increasing your speed, walking up hills, or walking with small hand weights. Always remember though to choose exercises that suit your fitness level. Particularly if you haven't done much physical activity in the past, be careful not to push yourself too hard, or too quickly.

Other great types of cardio include swimming, jogging, dancing, cycling and tennis. There are so many options and finding an exercise you love will make it far easier for it to become a part of your routine.

Aim for 30 minutes of low-impact cardio two to three days a week.

Here is a **Quick Morning Workout** idea to try:

I recommend starting the day with ten reps of five different exercises. So, if you can't do one of my workouts in your busy day, then this is a great way to start your day and kickstart that metabolism.

I have put these ideas together in a PDF for your download and stick to your fridge.

Go to www.50shadesofmenopause.co.uk to print yours out.

Here are some examples:

· Calf raises – lifting up onto your toes and lowering

· Tricep dips – on the floor or off a chair

· Knee lifts – raise your knee and lower the opposite elbow to it, alternating legs

· Squats – Press your bottom back as if you're going to sit on a chair. Keep your knees in line with your ankles, chest raised. Check your posture in the mirror if you're not sure or feel your knees are not positioned correctly.

· Squat kicks – Once you have your squat technique right you can try a squat then kick one leg out and alternate. This is great for balance, glute strength and cardio.

- A plank (held for the length of time you choose) — There are four plank positions to choose from so pick the position that works for you

- Press-ups (either off the kitchen counter or off the floor)

- Lunges — take a step forward into a bent knee (with the knee at 90 degrees) and step back to standing. The lower you go the harder it will be.

- Reverse lunges — the same as the forward lunge technique, but stepping backwards

- Jumping jacks — You can do these in a low-impact or high impact way to suit your own fitness level.

- Floor bridge — Lie on the floor on your back, legs hip-width apart, and raise your hips, squeezing your buttocks and then lower.

Choose five exercises and try doing ten repetitions of each. Make sure you mix it up each day to work different muscles and keep things interesting.

Visit the website www.50shadesofmenopause.co.uk for daily workout videos to follow and print out the PDF to help remind you to try some of these exercises.

All fitness levels are accommodated so I know you will find something that works for you and see how amazing you can feel in just a few days.

Remember exercise helps reduce symptoms of menopause, by helping you increase your metabolism, maintain a healthy weight, reduce stress, ease joint and muscle aches and pains, naturally balance hormones by releasing endorphins, serotonin and dopamine that counter low moods, all of which support our mental health and physical well-being.

What's not to love!

3. Nutrition

As discussed in Chapter 5 nutrition is a big subject and one that will make a huge difference to the way you feel throughout and beyond menopause.

Nutrition is so important that you will find a detailed nutrition guide on the website to guide you to making good food choices for your body and mind.

I also provide you with a 14-day meal plan to help get you started on eating properly, understanding good nutrition, and variations on foods that you may not have tried before or didn't realise you could eat.

The best way to look at food is as a source of energy. The body can only function in an optimal way if it has the right sources of energy going into it. Just think what happens if you accidentally put petrol into a car that uses diesel – it wrecks the engine and it won't work properly.

Similarly, if you eat lots of processed fast food, high sugar, high saturated fat foods, with no fruit or vegetables or nutrients, your body lacks energy and your body's organs and hormones can't function properly. You feel lethargic, you gain fat around your organs, tummy, waist and thighs, and you feel mentally drained.

When it comes to nutrition, I have six golden rules. Keeping these in mind can help make eating healthy far less daunting.

Six Golden Rules

Rule number one is that preparation is key

Create a healthy meal plan for your week and stick to it to avoid that impulsive takeaway or making other bad food decisions. In Chapter 5 we talked about the many benefits of making home-cooked meals, but if you struggle to fit this into your schedule, consider using your weekends to do some meal prep for the coming week.

Cut up vegetables ready to be used or store some frozen fruit in the freezer so you can throw together a healthy smoothie in the morning.

And just as you take the time to plan and prepare your meals, do the same for your snacks. Make sure you have healthy options in your fridge or pantry that you can reach for when hunger or cravings strike.

My daughter prepares carrot sticks and puts them in Tupperware to store in the fridge. Which means that when we want a sweet and tasty snack, they are there in the fridge ready to go. The fact they are crunchy and sweet really helps you feel satisfied and they're a great go-to snack for any time throughout your week.

Rule number two – fat does not make you fat!

Most women think that fats are bad and will add fat to your body, but this is not the case. They offer the body lots of energy, and there is a big difference between healthy fats and unhealthy saturated fats.

So, let's look at the positives that good fats offer the body. Good fat protects the internal organs, the subcutaneous fat, below the skin, helps insulate the body, plus it protects nerve endings. It helps transport vitamins A, D, E and K around the body for proper absorption. It helps regulate the menstrual cycle, it helps to suppress hunger and gives the feeling of being full. Stored body fat provides unlimited energy reserves when other nutrients aren't available.

So, what are healthy fats?

They are unsaturated fats that originate from plant sources and are generally liquid when they are at room temperature. Examples are avocados, peanuts, peanut oil, olive oil, soya beans, coconut oil and corn oils.

It is recommended that for the general population, the daily fat intake should be around 30% of the total energy intake.

Saturated fat (unhealthy fats) can be found in butter, cheese and fatty meats like beef, pork and lamb. These foods also have high cholesterol and can cause heart disease, strokes and cancers and are the cause of unhealthy weight gain. The other reason fat has such a bad reputation is that, in our Western diet, so many fatty foods are also combined with loads of sugar – and that's a sure-fire way to gain weight.

Which leads me into **rule number three**:

Stay away from sugar. By now, I'm sure I don't need to discuss the many reasons we need to cut sugar from our diets, but if you haven't done so already, go back and read to Chapter 5. The negative effects of sugar on the body are endless, and these are only exacerbated during menopause. That's why it's particularly important to cut as much sugar from your diet as possible.

Throughout the programme, I give you helpful tips to manage sugar cravings, and point you towards some healthy alternatives.

Rule number four ties in with another key element of the 21 Day Programme – **drink lots of water**.

As we discussed earlier in the chapter, drinking plenty of water makes it easier to lose weight, perform better in your workouts and will help you stay clear-headed throughout the day.

If you find water a bit dull on its own, try jazzing it up with a slice of lemon, lime or orange, or adding strawberries or cucumber to your glass.

Rule number five – keep alcohol to a minimum. The way the body processes alcohol is very similar to the way it processes sugar. Plus there are all the other negative health conditions alcohol can cause such as liver conditions, increased risk of heart disease and stroke, vitamin deficiency and a higher risk of cancer.

While a glass of wine once in a while is okay as a treat, make sure it's not a nightly occurrence and during the 21 day programme try not to indulge and give yourself a 21 day cleanse off alcohol.

Rule number six is arguably the most important, and that's to **listen to your body**. Pay attention to what causes your symptoms to flare up, what gives you energy and what makes you feel sluggish. Your journal is a great way to do this. But before you reach for a snack, also pay attention to whether or not you are actually hungry.

Is that hunger spike caused by a sudden drop in blood sugar that came as a result of eating something sweet? Are you thirsty and dehydrated? Are you stress eating to try and get rid of negative emotions? Or are you genuinely hungry?

Listen, learn and take action!

Portion Sizes

The amount of food you eat is just as important as what you eat, especially if you are struggling with your weight.

The amount of calories we should consume varies for each of us, depending on our weight, age and whether we want to maintain or lose weight, or build muscle.

As a broad figure, menopausal women should be consuming between 1500 and 2000 calories per day (this is all dependent on how active you are).

Working out the correct meal portions can be daunting, so here's an easy rule to follow to make sure you are eating the right amount, and making sure you're getting something from each important food group:

Aim to fill one quarter of your plate with proteins such as lean meat, fish, beans or pulses. Fill one quarter of the plate with healthy fats, such as avocado, egg or nuts. Fill one quarter with vegetables and the remaining quarter with complex carbohydrates brown rice, sweet potato or brown pasta.

Your protein source (meat and fish) should be approximately the size of your open palm, and aim for your carb source (potato, pasta, rice etc) to be around the size of your cupped hand.

If you are trying to lose weight, however, I recommend replacing the carbohydrates with more fruits or vegetables. And if you want to gain muscle, then increase the amount of lean protein.

What exactly is protein?

Many women know that protein-rich diets are very popular at the moment, but don't really know why. I'm going to break down exactly what protein does for you, so you can understand this a little more clearly.

Protein is essential for a multitude of bodily functions related to growth, maintenance and repair. Proteins are made up of amino acids which are the building blocks for every living cell in the body including the skin, muscles, tendons, ligaments, hair, bones and teeth.

There are 20 amino acids that make up protein. The body produces ONLY 12 of these and the rest are found in dietary sources.

If you are not eating a good diet of fruit and vegetables, then your body is not getting the essential amino acids it needs to function optimally. Without the right amount of amino acids absorbed the body will generate the energy it needs from protein found in muscle and organ tissues. This is not what you want as it depletes muscle instead of building it.

You can find protein in all meat, fish and dairy. It is also found in vegetables, pulses and legumes.

We need to maintain good protein levels in our bodies during menopause as it helps keep up our energy levels, it helps with regulating hormone changes, and it helps to maintain and build muscles. Protein also helps to produce antibodies which help us resist viruses and illness.

A normal daily diet should be around 10-12% protein, which is enough to give you your daily energy. If you are resistance training then this can go up slightly to 15% so that your body can maintain, recover and rebuild.

What are carbohydrates?

Carbohydrates are the body's preferred source of energy. When the body breaks carbohydrates down, it forms glucose, which the body in turn uses for energy.

There are two types of carbohydrates. There are simple carbohydrates which are usually referred to as simple sugars and include refined sugars like cake, chocolate and biscuits.

CHAPTER SEVEN:

These often provide the body with empty calories and can be known as "free" sugars. This means the body cannot find any good use for the food, and unless it can use the energy it will be stored as fat in the body.

Simple sugars can also be natural, such as those found in fruit. These carbohydrates have essential vitamins and minerals required by the body to function as micro-nutrients.

There are also complex carbohydrates which are often recognised as starches and found in potatoes, brown rice, brown pasta and porridge. Complex carbohydrates take longer to digest and so provide a longer source of energy.

The main use of carbohydrates is energy. The brain and nervous system use the energy from blood glucose to function effectively.

Carbohydrates also have a muscle sparing effect, which means they prevent the body using muscle protein as a source of energy. This helps to maintain a healthy metabolism and keeps energy levels available for organs and skeletal muscle, which consume large amounts of energy each day.

I advise women to exercise with resistance and weights, it's to increase their skeletal muscle, which thereby increases their metabolisms. It also helps to lower adipose tissue (fat) stores, which are energy stores created by simple carbohydrates (sugars).

Dietary fibre is the name given to plant-based carbohydrates like whole grains, cereals and fruit. These are important for optimal digestive health because these carbohydrates help to transport food and waste matter through the gastrointestinal tract.

Dietary fibre can be both soluble and insoluble. Soluble fibre is found in oat bran, barley, nuts, seeds, beans, lentils, peas and some fruits and vegetables.

Insoluble fibre is found in wheat bran, vegetables and whole grains. This is what bulks food and helps your stools pass through the digestive system. Not enough of either type of dietary fibre can cause constipation.

Healthy Fats

We need healthy unsaturated fats for our bodies to use as stored energy. If you have been on diets in the past, then you have probably been told that fats are bad for you and that you should remove fats from your diet. This is incorrect.

The truth is we need to remove saturated fats which harmfully clog our arteries and can cause heart disease. Fats found in fast food, chips, microwave meals, processed foods, cakes and treats are the fats you need to remove.

But healthy fats from foods like unsalted cashews, pistachios, peanuts, almonds, walnuts, avocado, mackerel, kippers, flaxseed and chia seeds, are fats that the body can use to help satiate your appetite leave you feeling full and give you energy for effective muscle and organ use.

Within the nutrition guide it maps out everything you need to know about what fruits, vegetables, fridge and pantry essentials will be best for you. This is not a diet it is a way of re-learning what food will support you and not trigger menopause symptoms whilst also being tasty and nutritious.

Maintaining a balanced diet where you know the quantity of protein, healthy fats and carbohydrates will really help to manage weight and adipose tissue during menopause.

As we age, we have to be considerate of what our bodies need and how the energy we eat is being used. One of the key points here is that calorie counting and trying to eat less is **not** the goal.

The goal is to feel more energised, to use the calories and energy we consume and thereby not add weight to our tummies, hips and thighs, which are the areas we are more prone to holding weight during menopause.

The foods in the meal plan help to optimise hormones levels, reduce inflammation and detoxify the body.

Foods to Boost Your Metabolism

I've mentioned about our metabolisms dropping as we age, but there are a great range of superfoods that will help boost it. I've included these as part of your daily meal plan. So, let's quickly look at what they can do for you:

Let's start with flaxseed. Flaxseed is a phytoestrogen, which helps lift oestrogen levels and promote hormone balance.

It helps increase energy, reduces fat and improves glucose levels.

A study found that eating flaxseed decreased hot flashes in menopause by 60%. Flaxseed oil is a polyunsaturated fatty acid and is an anti-inflammatory. It has been used to treat rheumatoid arthritis, is packed with omega-3 and fatty acids to help detoxify your system.

Ginger root is another great superfood. It helps decrease inflammation in the gut and stimulates digestion. It can also act as an appetite suppressant.

Studies show that ginger can increase metabolism in animals by 20%. It has around 40 antioxidant properties that prevent free radical damage and protect against aging. It also improves skin elasticity for a more youthful appearance.

Lentils are a rich source of complex carbohydrates; a nutrient that boosts the metabolism and helps burn body fat. They are high in fibre and magnesium, which also helps reduce inflammation in the gut. They are rich in folic acid, which helps to balance hormones.

Lentils provide antioxidant vitamins A and C which again help protect against free radicals. They're great for detoxification.

Avocados are rich in healthy fats that are proven to boost metabolism. Research has shown that people who eat avocados have less belly fat than those who don't. They are a healthy source of monounsaturated fat and antioxidants that relieve inflammation. They also help ease the symptoms of multiple sclerosis.

Avocados balance cholesterol and the stress hormone cortisol. They contain 14 grams of fibre which helps the removal of toxins and reduces premature aging.

Cinnamon is an anti-inflammatory sweet spice that helps fight infection and repairs tissue. It's an amazing anti-aging spice. Research shows a link between cinnamon and increased metabolism. It's seen as a powerhouse spice that can aid changes in the body at a cellular level.

These superfoods can have an amazing effect on increasing your metabolic rate, reducing inflammation in the body, detoxifying the body and helping your hormones become more balanced. They also aid in weight management and stress relief.

As you can no doubt see, good nutrition is hugely important during menopause, just as it is throughout your life.

Head over to www.50shadesofmenopause.co.uk for the meal plan and nutrition guide to get started

4. Sleep

The importance of sleep is often completely underestimated. When we don't have enough sleep, our bodies aren't able to re-charge and recover. Lack of sleep leaves us feeling tired, groggy headed, fatigued, lacklustre, headachy, intolerant of people and situations and we can struggle to handle normal day-to-day tasks.

Menopause insomnia and hot flashes can occur in the early hours of the morning breaking sleep and leaving you feeling drained and out of sorts throughout your day. Lots of things can trigger poor sleep during menopause. Spicy food, caffeine, stress, hormone fluctuations, lack of exercise and too much sugar are all culprits.

It's important to develop good sleep hygiene methods to ease symptoms and get your body into a better sleeping pattern. Think back to when you were a child, you probably had a good 'before bedtime' routine created by your parents to help you go to bed and sleep.

You probably would have had a set time to go upstairs, either to have a calming bath or to have a bedtime story and then lights out would be consistently at the same.

As adults we have too many choices. Most of the time we have created our own habits of sitting down in an evening and mindlessly watching whatever is on the TV, while at the same time checking our social media apps and reviewing what to buy next from a popular online store.

The blue light from our computer screens, TVs and phones are not good for us in an evening as it stimulates the brain when it should be easing into sleep mode.

Instead of allowing the brain to be lulled into a restful state, we pump it up with adrenaline by watching an exciting drama or thriller. The blue light we stare into engages our brain cells to trigger ideas and process new things when we really should be calming it down at the end of the day.

So… what can we do to help our sleep patterns now we are in menopause?

Sleep hygiene is all about finding an extra half an hour to an hour of sleep a night to help us balance our hormones and ease our stress levels. It's about getting rid of those bad habits, like staring at the TV screen or social media until the moment we try to sleep.

Instead, try doing something to relax yourself before going to bed. Taking a bath or meditating, reading a good book or doing a crossword can help to calm the mind and prepare for sleep.

If you are particularly stressed try writing in your journal to brain dump all your worries and concerns there, so they don't replay over and over in your mind causing you to wake up anxious or become restless during the night.

Keep distracting things like your phone and TV out of the bedroom, and avoid anything moderately stimulating, such as exercise, watching movies, or using the computer in the hour before you go to bed.

Consistency is key. Aim to go to bed at the same time each night. As ladies in my programme can attest to, the week-ends are often the hardest times to stick to new habits, so it's particularly important that you keep to your sleep schedule on Friday and Saturday nights if you can. And though it might be tempting to lounge around in bed all day after a night of tossing and turning and hot flashes, the best thing you can do is to get up at the same time every day.

Remember you are going to try this for 21 days to start getting your body and mind into a new routine. Once you consistently get that extra half an hour of sleep a night, the benefits of feeling more refreshed during the day with less menopause anxiety and stress will make it completely worthwhile sticking to.

5. Self-Care

As women we are carers for others. It's in our DNA to look after children, work colleagues, family, the home, our parents and friends.

On a normal daily list of things to do I'm sure, like me, you put all the things you would really like to do for yourself at the bottom of the list. Or you just don't add them in at all!

The idea of self-care is foreign to most of us, but with the 21 Day Programme, allotting a small pocket of your day to doing something that makes you smile is essential to managing your menopause.

In the programme, I ask you to plan in just 15 - 20 minutes per day for doing something that is related to making you feel better; something that will help you manage your menopause journey with a little more control and will make you smile!

Unfortunately, for many of us, putting time aside for self-care leads us to feeling guilty. All too often, we associate self-care with being indulgent or selfish, when in reality it's essential for mental health and wellness.

I am a great believer that if you want to be there for your family and friends, the best thing you can do is be there for yourself first.

Self-care can look different for everyone, but it's all about finding that precious "Me" time and scheduling it into your day. Yes, that's right – schedule it in, because for most of us, it's the only way of getting it done.

Start thinking about the things you love to do. Is there something that you used to love doing that you no longer find time for because life got in the way?

Think about creating a self-care list – a list of all the things you would like to do, just for yourself.

It might include simple things like buying yourself flowers, burning your favourite essential oils, or spending time in the garden.

Maybe you'd like to have a massage, go to a museum or take a drive to a place you've always wanted to go. Maybe it's about getting up ten minutes earlier each day to meditate or allowing yourself to have a nap in the afternoon.

One of the best self-care methods I've found since teaching Pilates and finding meditation is how fantastic breathing techniques are to help calm the mind and ease stress.

Here are two techniques that help you calm down during the day and can also help ease yourself to sleep at night:

Breathing Techniques

The first is the "**deep breath sniff**" technique, that I like to use during the day. This can be done sitting in a chair, or cross-legged on the floor or lying in bed.

Close your eyes, relax your body, unclench your jaw. Take a deep breath in and hold it for a moment. Then take another sniff of breath in, before slowly letting the breath go. Make sure you exhale fully and then repeat.

Repeat this 3, to 5 times to start feeling the benefit.

The second breathing exercise I love is the "**four-count breath**" exercise. It's a great one to help yourself relax before you go to sleep each night. Either lying down or sitting, with your eyes closed, inhale deeply through the nose for a count of four, hold for four and then exhale slowly through the mouth for the count of four.

Again, do this at least 3 times to feel the benefit. I find this is a great way to help me drop off to sleep.

Priming

Another self-care exercise I love, and one that I recommend my clients do each day is Priming. This is a great way to get yourself centred and ready to take on the day ahead. Do this exercise either sitting cross-legged if it's comfortable for you or seated in a chair.

Close your eyes and think about something that makes you smile. This might be the memory of a holiday you've been on, something somebody said to you, or maybe a pet you love. Alternatively, you can imagine yourself in a time and place in which you felt most special and good about yourself.

Hold your arms above your head, deeply inhale, exhale whilst bringing your arms down quickly, bending at the elbow to shoulder height. Inhale and raise your arms, exhale and lower your arms, bending at the elbow, and repeat quickly. Do this 20 times, as quickly as you can.

Once you have completed the 20 inhalation and exhalations, sit calmly with your eyes closed and your hands on your lap, palms facing upwards. Feel your heartbeat and the tingling in your hands that comes from your body taking in all that oxygen.

As you sit quietly with your eyes closed, tell yourself that you are going to have a great day. Know that whatever challenges life throws your way, it is something you are able to handle it with a smile.

There's a video on the website demonstrating this so you know what it looks and feels like.

This is a great way to set yourself up for a positive day, reduce anxiety, improve confidence, boost your energy by actively moving your arms up and down quickly and using your breath to focus.

Metabolism Boosting Cold Showers

In my most recent programme, we added in a 10-20 second blast of cold water to the end of your daily shower.

Shower as normal and at the end just turn the cold water on for 10-20 seconds to energise you before getting out.

The cold water stimulates your metabolism to kickstart and work at a higher-than-normal energy-burning level. As I have mentioned several times throughout the book, lifting your metabolic rate daily will increase your energy and thereby improve the way the body handles hormones, aging and menopause.

Under the cold water, the blood in your body races to your major organs, flooding them with oxygenated blood and as you get out of the shower the blood then floods back to your extremities, feeding your skin cells and muscles.

Ice baths have long been used by athletes to reduce muscle tears, lessen muscle soreness and improve injury recovery. Supporters of cold-water therapy believe that cold water can improve your circulation, deepen your sleep, spike your energy levels and reduce inflammation in your body.

Therefore, when ending your shower, why not try a cooling boost of energy from the cold tap?

Have a Massage

We all know that a massage feels great, and studies have shown that getting a massage not only helps relax muscles, but it also helps reduce cortisol levels – the stress hormone that likes to wreak havoc on our bodies.

Whatever you choose as your self-care practise, make sure it's in line with the rest of the elements in the 21 Day Programme. Above all, allow yourself to take this time without feeling guilty, as you deserve to feel good about yourself.

Keep in mind your hormone body type

In Chapter 2 you learnt about hormone body types. Keep these in mind when applying these new habits.

If you are more prone to being an adrenal or oestrogen body type, then you know that stress and cortisol need to be kept under control.

Focusing on exercises like Pilates, deep breathing, priming and Flow & Go on days you feel stressed is the best way to see results. Heavy strength workouts on these days will add stress rather than ease it. Try and recognise when you feel under pressure and try and find ways to self soothe and relax.

If the Liver Body Type feels more like you, then remember that you need to keep away from dairy as it will inflame your gut and slow down digestion.

Also, it would be better to do your workout early in the morning to help lift a low mood and ease yourself into a more positive day. Strength building workouts will help to stimulate your metabolism and boost your energy and strength levels.

If you are a Thyroid Body Type, make sure you have your thyroid checked regularly to maintain balance. Again, your energy levels will feel low if you have an under active thyroid so manage stress as best you can, long walks and toning exercises within Pilates and yoga will help.

As you know one size does not fit all with menopause. Learn what works for you and by journaling your progress you will be able to tweak your routine to make it one you enjoy following.

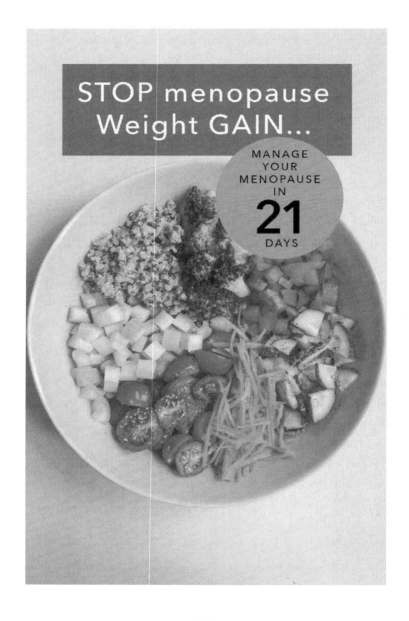

STOP menopause Weight GAIN...

MANAGE
YOUR
MENOPAUSE
IN
21
DAYS

CHAPTER EIGHT:

21 DAYS – LET'S GO!

'A woman is like a tea bag — you never know how strong she is until she gets in hot water.' – Eleanor Roosevelt

Throughout this book, I've given you facts about menopause and how it affects your body and mind so that you are ready to start your own 21-day menopause programme to reset yourself and feel heaps better.

Remember this is a starting point. Within less than 21 days you will feel many symptoms ease and possibly disappear, however the idea is to use this as your starting point to creating new healthier habits that will sustain you through all three stages of menopause.

You now know the fundamentals and the underlying triggers that cause your hormones to spike and menopause symptoms to become overwhelming.

So, now is the time to start getting excited. Now is the time to plan forward to ensure you have success. Now is the time to get your family and friends on board to support you managing your menopause in 21 days.

While I'd love for you to join me on my next 21 Day Programme, you will get great results on your own by following this simple daily plan:

DAILY PLAN TO STICK TO FOR 21 DAYS

HEAD SPACE

Get positive especially first thing in the morning.

Create an 'I can do this' mantra to get yourself revved up and ready for your day

Plan, plan, plan for success, look at your notes and what you are going to do to make today work for you.

Go to the website and follow the Priming video for your daily morning pep up.

Go to the appendix in this book and read your morning daily message.

This is your time. You are going to feel amazing in the next 3-4 days and beyond - just take the first step.

WATER

Start each day with a large glass of water to rehydrate your body and mind before eating or drinking anything else.

Make it something you enjoy by adding a slice of lemon or fresh fruit like strawberries, cherries, cucumber. Avoid sugary squashes and fruit juices these are a "no-no", throughout the whole of the programme.

During the day try and drink a glass of water at mid-morning, lunchtime and mid-afternoon. This will hydrate your cells and clear your mind. Again, you can add fruit to help detoxify your body or try an un-caffeinated herbal tea.

To help you remember to drink regularly during your day use a lovely alarm on your phone to remind you, until it becomes a habit. You are aiming for 8 glasses of water a day.

End the day with a large mug of hot water.

NUTRITION

Go to the website and download the Meal Plan and shopping guide. Buy everything you need for your first week ahead of time. And remove unhealthy foods from your fridge and pantry that will possibly trip you up.

The meals are tasty, filling, with a few snack options that means you won't feel like you are on a diet and will help you cope with moments of weakness in a healthy way.

Remember we are creating a new way of life so start to enjoy the process and get your family to enjoy it with you.

Reduce your caffeine intake by choosing decaffeinated tea or coffee and reduce the number of cups you have in a day.

Avoid alcohol.

Choose smaller portions, use the palm of the hand rule for your protein and carbohydrates (there is a video on the website for you to watch about portion control that will help), eat as many vegetables (especially greens) as you want.

Don't eat later than 7pm at night. Give your body chance to digest before bedtime.

Keep it simple, eat three meals a day and make sure you feel full after each meal.

EXERCISE

Plan in a 15-20 minute walk every day. Plan in exercise and movement as it is not necessarily something you do naturally at the start and will be the first thing you will avoid doing if you have a busy day!

Starting the day with a walk is a great way to energise your mind and body and reduce aches.

Do a 10 – 20-minute workout each day and mix up what you do. Go to the website for a range of workouts to choose from. There's Pilates for flexibility, strength and calmness; low-impact aerobics to help burn fat.Enjoy the strength training at least 2 times in your week – you can use cans to start and move on to hand weights when you feel more confident.

Building good muscle tone will raise your metabolism, give you more energy naturally between workouts and reduce adipose tissue around your tummy.

During the 21 days try and exercise six days a week and rest for the seventh day. You will see your energy levels rise and you will feel more confident and become stronger.

Always workout to your level and if you have any underlying health issues, please see your doctor for advice before starting. Most importantly your body will feel less achy and sore, and you will start to sleep better.

SELF-CARE

Take time out each day to do something for yourself. Read a book, learn something new, meditate, breathe deeply, go for that walk to clear your head.

Find what makes you smile and do it, even if it's only for a short space of time like a 10-minute block.

You will see over the days how much easier it gets to put yourself first but also how much calmer you feel and more fulfilled with life.

JOURNAL

On the website there's access to a Journal that you can download and use as a guide to know what to write if you want guidance.

Get to know yourself.

Each day, write down how you feel when you wake up and what your previous day held that might have affected how you slept and feel on waking.

How are your symptoms?

Did you do something to self-sabotage your day the day before? if so, what are you going to do today to avoid the same issue happening.

Did you have a headache from coming off the caffeine?

Know that every day is a new day and that you can take back control over your actions.

Start looking at what symptoms are easing over the 21 days to know you are feeling better.

Recognise how amazing you are and tell yourself you are "*enough*" and that "*you are worth it*".

SLEEP

Go to bed half an hour earlier than normal (an hour if you can). Make sure you have no blue light equipment such as a TV, phone or laptop near you for at least 30 minutes if not an hour before lights off.

Create a lovely habit for going to bed and making yourself feel nice and calm. Do this consistently for the 21 days, including the weekend.

Remember how important sleep is for repair, recovery and balancing your hormones. If you need help with sleeping use the breathing techniques in Chapter 7 or find a sleep app on your phone with some calming meditation or white noise to help ease your mind into a deep sleep.

CHAPTER EIGHT:

Look at Chapter 8 every day, to remind yourself of each step.

Also make sure you go to the appendix and get your daily positive message from me to give yourself a pep up for the day ahead.

Most importantly have fun doing the 21 days. Everything you need can be found on www.50shadesofmenopause.co.uk.

Small Steps forward each day will lead you to success. So don't give up and instead, keep your mental attitude strong and willing.

Choose to enjoy the process and you will start to find everything easier to follow after the first 4 days and will want to continue to see more results.

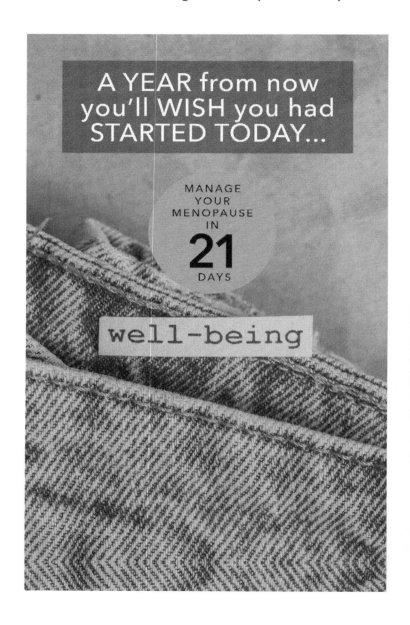

A YEAR from now you'll WISH you had STARTED TODAY...

MANAGE YOUR MENOPAUSE IN

21

DAYS

well-being

CONCLUSION

'During menopause oestrogen drops and cortisol rises'

There you have it... a clear road map to follow for 21 days to re-find the old you!

Some of these new habits may feel a little tricky to add into your daily routine at first, but it's all about planning forward, taking small steps each day and over time those habits become your normal way of life.

Know that each day is a new day to reset and restart. Use each morning to start with the right intentions. You can recalibrate how you handle stressful situations. Creating new fall-back tips and tricks to help stop self-sabotage and keep you on track. Everything you do within the 21 Days is going to help you learn about your body and mind.

You'll start to love your new heathier habits and find them easier to stick to as the results become apparent. They will become something that you do more often than not to create a new balance in your life.

In 21-days you will see amazing changes to your body and an easing of your menopause symptoms, but remember it is a starting point for you. It takes a little time for the new habits to be taken on board so that they remain with you for the rest of your life.

What you can often find is that once you finish the 21 Day Programme, one of the five elements gives way. The planning forward may stop on meal prep and good nutrition. Or you might find that you have a busy week, and the exercise goes out of the window. Or you don't plan in your daily walk.

Keeping up your sleep hygiene and having a regular bedtime routine can sometimes seem less important as you aren't accountable to anyone except yourself.

What happens when habits are not embedded is that your brain can easily talk you into going back to what used to feel comfortable, and that's where diets and quick result programmes fall down.

Don't let this happen to you.

When you have completed the 21 Day Menopause Programme, there is also a "Fit-For-Life" Maintenance Programme I offer to help keep you on track, so that the new habits embed themselves and stay with you.

There is more normality and ease to the maintenance programme which means that you are on a 5:2 protocol; this means five days of sticking to clean eating and two days for a little wiggle room with your nutrition and 3-4 workouts per week.

This should be so much easier after you complete the 21 days as it means you have a little bit of fluidity and flexibility to your week.

You will still need to plan, and you still need to make sure you have everything in place in order to move forward with ease, but once it becomes a habit then it is happily fixed in you.

Some of my ladies have been with me for over eight months after the initial 21 days and have maintained the results they obtained and continued to improve.

The aim in maintenance is to find balance. You can't always be looking for weight loss; you need to find a time and space to recognise that you are happy and have control over the things that felt out of control before.

We all have external things happen to us that can push us off track, including stressful things like Covid, bad news, job loss, bereavement, family stress, natural dips in our hormones and other irregular things that happen to our bodies during the menopause. It is much easier to handle them when you are maintaining good protocols.

We all need to take a first step towards helping ourselves. Try and think about what that means to you and what you will get from helping yourself right now.

When you're happy then everyone around you is happy. Happiness comes from a feeling of love; feeling like you have a little control over the uncontrollable (in this case the menopause) and knowing you're doing the best for yourself.

The menopause is a journey; and it's one that takes years. With this programme you will be guided to finding balance, getting stronger, losing belly fat, regaining energy and improving your sleep and stress levels.

So, what are you waiting for – get started today!

Go to www.50shadesofmenopause.co.uk download the meal plans and nutrition guide. Checkout the priming, workouts and journal and plan your next 21 days.

On a daily basis use the Appendix where you will find a daily message to keep you on track and motivate you to keep going.

You've totally got this and if you need any additional help or support you can email me at, hello@50shadesofmenopause .co.uk or you can join in on my next 21-day Manage Your Menopause Program.

You can also join my 50 Shades of Menopause Facebook group where you will find women like you, on the same journey, who are supportive and encouraging and will also make you laugh!!

Know that with a little determination and resolve, you will be capable of making the changes you need to not only navigate menopause, but to also live a healthy and happy life for many years to come.

CONCLUSION

You've totally got this!

Now go and smash it!

Best wishes,
Ailsa x

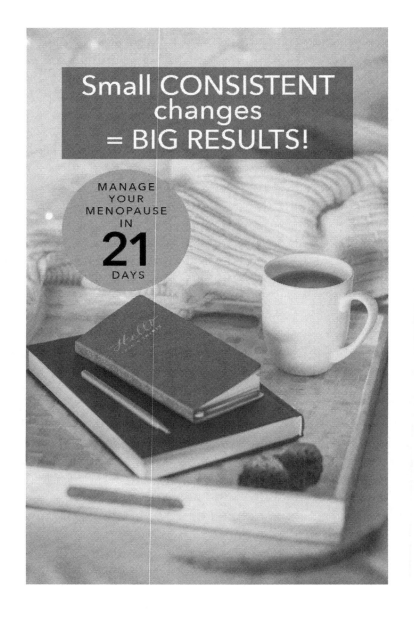

APPENDIX:

DAILY MESSAGES

' There are only 2 choices, make progress or make excuses'

Each morning of my 21 Day Menopause Programme, my ladies receive a positive message to boost their motivation and help them stay on track.

It's one of the elements of the programme that my clients find the most useful. As Marieke says:

"I have just completed Ailsa's 21 Day Menopause Programme, a combination of healthy eating, daily exercise, mindfulness, good sleep and drinking lots of water… Over three weeks I have seen an enormous difference: lost 8lbs and cm's all over, but most importantly, I feel so much better in myself. Brighter and clearer in my head, and more positive and motivated. And because of family circumstances I wasn't even able to follow the programme to the letter!

I am more determined than ever to keep going and to put myself first and be fit and healthy well into old age. I can't recommend this enough!"

As you work through the programme, you might find it useful to read a message each day from me, to help keep your spirits high.

So here we go!

DAY 1

Good Morning Day 1!

I hope you feel prepared and excited to make some positive changes! We all need to feel like we're not alone and so please know that we're all going through this together.

Here are a few helpful tips to get your journey off to the right start:

1. Start every day with a glass of water before you do anything else.

2. Schedule in a daily walk. You can do this first thing in the morning, during your lunch break, or as a distraction for cravings.

3. Reduce, if not cut out caffeine. If that sounds like a struggle, go decaf to start, but try to stop at one cup as it dehydrates you and will add to your current symptoms.

4. Try to cut out sugar and stick to healthy, clean eating. You'll find everything you need in the Meal Plans and Nutrition Guide on the website and go back to Chapter 7 for reminders.

5. Plan in your exercise. If you haven't done your Fitness Test then do it today. Follow the exercise demonstrations to find alternatives and always workout to your fitness level. Exercise is best done in the morning if you can as you have more energy and it will give you energy for your day ahead.

6. Drink lots of water throughout your day.

7. Take some 'Me' time to breathe, so you can keep your mindset positive and strong.

8. Plan your bedtime. Try and go to bed half an hour earlier than normal, plan a lovely bedtime routine to calm your mind and get you into a better headspace to sleep.

9. Keep a positive mindset and know that once you get past the first three days it will all start to feel easier.

In less than 21 days you are going to be feeling amazing!

So, here's to a fantastic first day − it's all about planning ahead and not letting your mind distract you back to your normal habits.

If you do get cravings, move and get active, clean your teeth, do a workout, go for a walk or drink water. Cravings only last four minutes and distraction and action is the key to overcoming them.

You've totally got this! Have the best day.

DAY 2

Good morning and congratulations, you got through Day 1! You're on your way. How did you find it?

Make sure you write in your journal how you feel when you wake up and any symptoms you're dealing with. Check in with yourself to start the day strong!

Don't forget to re-look at what your goals are and focus on those as it helps to keep you energised and on track.

Today, it's all about small consistent steps that will reap big changes. Know that you'll see the rewards across your entire body and mind as you go through the programme, and this will help you build new, healthier, long-lasting habits.

Today, make sure you plan your meals ahead of time so you know what you're eating. Don't just leave it to chance, follow the meal plan as closely as you can. Keep the clean eating mindset and momentum and you'll start to feel the results, starting with your head space.

Day 2 is a great time to start practising Priming. Have a go at Priming in the mornings to set yourself up for the day ahead. This will help energise you, and gets you thinking positively – plus it feels amazing! (Refer to Chapter 7 on self-care for how to do it plus go the www.50shadesofmenopause.co.uk for a demonstration.)

Don't forget to start the day with water to keep you hydrated and clear your head. This is especially important first thing in the morning but also throughout your day.

And don't forget our craving avoidance techniques: Remember, a craving only lasts four minutes, so any time it strikes, move from the place you are sitting and get active. You can also try cleaning your teeth, as nothing tastes great with toothpaste or when your mouth feels clean!

And if you have to have anything, go for chopped sticks of carrots or cucumber (look at the meal plan for guidance on small snacks if you need them and only stick to those suggestions).

It's all a case of mind over matter at this stage – but I know you can do it!

The first three days are all about removing processed foods from your body. It takes 72 hours to fully clear your body of processed foods as they slow down your digestion, so by Day 4 you'll feel a lot better both mentally and physically – just stick with it!

Have the best Day 2 – take a moment today to focus on one positive thing that happened recently. This will do wonders for your mindset!

You've totally got this.

DAY 3

Good morning, it's Day 3 already! If you struggle with cravings, you will possibly still be feeling them today – that's totally normal. Just keep using that amazing willpower to go for healthy options. You may also feel headachy from caffeine withdrawal but keep drinking water and you'll start feeling a lift to that very soon.

You've totally got this – remember today might be the one that feels a little tricky. This can be due to a number of things: Firstly, your brain will always want to revert to what it knows and go back to old habits. This is why on Day 3 you'll experience that little realisation that you're doing something different.

Secondly, remember your body is still digesting any processed foods in your system. If you're feeling sluggish, it's likely related to that, along with a slower gut response. But stay on track – just wait and see how much better you're going to feel tomorrow and onwards.

Thirdly, you are now exercising and walking on a daily basis but for many of us, it's not a habit yet, so your brain may say *"not interested today!"* But push through, plan in your workout and just do it anyway!

Enjoy your day – remember to plan those meals and really stick to it as you'll start seeing some nice changes tomorrow and moving forward.

DAY 4

Yay it's Day 4! How are you feeling? Are you journaling and getting to know yourself a little better?

I hope you're making notes in your journals daily of how you're feeling when you wake up and if any foods are agreeing or disagreeing with you, plus any symptoms that are starting to ease or have popped up unexpectedly! You'll be surprised after the 21 days about where you started and how far you have progressed.

What have been the tricky moments for you and what did you do to help avoid slipping into your normal routine? When you know what to do to make small changes to your daily habits, it will help you break through from what has been holding you back.

Don't forget your morning water and if you've been sticking to the meal plan and reducing /or removing caffeine from your day, then from today onwards your body is going to really start feeling the benefits.

The headaches and lethargy will lift and you will start to not crave sugar in the same way as you did, because you've reduced it right out of your meals. This is going to have such a positive impact on you and your hormones and your symptoms.

Today, think about doing a body conditioning workout – we need to get the strength building back into your bodies. You can use either cans or light hand weights. It'll lift your endorphins, lift your cardio and strengthen those muscles.

Have the best day. You are over halfway through this first week. Be sure to stick with it as you're going to start to see and feel some really positive changes.

Keep strong, you're smashing it!

DAY 5

How are you all doing? It's Day 5!

If you started the programme on a Monday, today will be a prep day for your weekend. The key to this first weekend is to stay on track – your natural relief that it's the weekend is linked to your normal habits of snacking and eating probably a less healthy menu of food.

To get on top of this, I need you to do a good shop for healthy snacks so you don't feel tempted to fall off the wagon! You'll find that in a few days you'll start to see some proper easing of your symptoms, and if you've been sticking to the meal plan and the workouts, you're going to be feeling much better.

Your body will be more energised and starting to get used to the variety of exercises you're doing easing stiffness, joint pain and starting to tone and build cardio and muscle strength!

Please keep making your journal notes to keep track of your progress you should be feeling proud of yourself for reaching Day 5 already.

How is your sleep hygiene going? Are you making sure you're trying to get to bed that ½ an hour earlier? Are you putting your phone down and stopping social media a little earlier than usual?

If so you'll be starting to build up the benefits of the extra sleep time and the better quality sleep, which will notice-ably change your head space through the day to being more positive. Make your night-time routine so lovely you can't wait to go to bed.

Don't forget to drink lots of water – this should become a little mantra in your head!

I hope you have the best day and feel proud that you have got to Day 5.

It's awesome and another day of turning that corner and being kind to yourself. If you haven't already, you'll soon start to feel your sluggishness ease along with those detox headaches.

You've totally got this!

DAY 6

Woohoo it's Day 6 and you're doing amazingly well! If you started the programme on a Monday, it's the weekend to-day, so please try and maintain your new routine.

REMEMBER:

Drink a big glass of water when you wake up and keep drinking throughout your day to stay alert and energised.

Have three clean meals. Use the meal plan to know what you'll be eating and look forward to feeling full and energised from the tasty selections on there.

Enjoy a calming walk, no matter what the weather! I love walking when it's cold and snowy and when no one is around. The cold air in my face feels so freeing! In the Summer, it's lovely to go out really early before the heat of the day and see all the colour around you. If you stop and take a photo on your walk it really keeps you in the moment and you can appreciate the beauty around you.

Don't forget your workout. Put on your own music and enjoy strengthening the body and balancing your hormones.

Don't forget to try Priming if you haven't already. It's a great way to reset your day at any time – so if you feel bleh go and do five minutes of Priming to lift your mood.

Make sure to schedule some "Me" time into your day. Plan ahead to give yourself 10, 15, 30 or 60 mins of time today to do something to makes you smile and breathe – you deserve it!

Weekend or not, try and maintain that better sleep routine. You'll feel much better with an extra 30 minutes of sleep.

The weekend is the perfect time to relax after a busy week but it does give you time to fall into old habits. The last thing we want is to sabotage all the good stuff we've been doing. If you feel your old habits trying to take over, fight them and choose a healthy option this weekend. You'll be so pleased you did when you see how you feel next week.

Remember to make notes in your journal. The weekend is a great time to take a look back at your week and see how you felt when you started this journey. Note down any changes – both good and bad – to help you understand yourself.

Remember to take it a day at a time. Don't look too far ahead – even the smallest steps forward will take you where you want to go.

Have the best day – you've totally got this!

DAY 7

Well done, you've done a full week! How are you feeling?!

Day 7 on the programme is scheduled as a rest day, but that only means a rest from doing a proper workout. So, firstly be honest with yourself. If you have missed any workout days this week, use today to add it back in! Just get that extra workout done – you'll feel so proud of yourself that you did.

If you have done a workout every day so far, do have a rest, but make sure you enjoy a dance around the kitchen! It's fun, uplifting and something you can have a giggle doing.

Today is about celebrating YOU. Be proud that you've stuck to the programme. It's important to recognise how well you're doing and how far you've come.

Write down in your journal how you feel today, how your symptoms are, whether you're feeling better, whether you still have cravings, and if so, when they happen. Are they just old habits we need to help you quash? Also recognise and own up to yourself about any blips and think of ways not to get caught out by them in the week ahead.

If you have stuck to most of the programme – especially the exercise and clean eating – you will be starting to really feel and notice some results, so please stick with it today.

The celebration drink is water. The celebration treat is fruit. The energy booster is to dance around the kitchen, the mindfulness time is doing something to make you feel good – and don't forget to breathe deep, enjoy the moment and sleep.

You're awesome!

DAY 8

Good morning my lovely, here we are at Day 8!

You've got through the first week – and the first weekend woohoo! The weekends can be tough as the small routines we have during the middle of the week are not there to help us stay on track.

As we talked about yesterday, if you have a blip then own it. Write about it in your journal and make today a great day for returning to clean eating and ensure you get that exercise into your day. No self-sabotage or guilt is needed – just a positive head space. Instead of criticising yourself, work out how to avoid another blip today.

Don't forget to start your day with a big glass of water and a little Priming to get your mindset on point. Doing a core workout today is a great way to strengthen those abs.

Follow the Meal Plan for Day 8-14. New recipes to try and make sure you keep the variety of new food going.

Have the best day and know this week is going to feel amazing. As each day passes you'll feel some lovely changes start to show.

You've totally got this.

DAY 9

Good morning ladies, I'm hoping you are all feeling good. This week is about consistency and sticking to what you've been doing. You are past the toughest phase of the first week, which is so awesome; now it's about creating new healthier habits so the changes you have started to include in your daily life are habits that stick.

Forming a new habit is all about consistently doing something over a sustained period of time.

So, keep the strengthening exercises going and keep drinking water. Keep up the clean eating, keep practicing mindfulness and keep up that new sleep routine. If you do, you will start seeing a clearer head space, your emotions may feel more manageable and far less like an emotional rollercoaster! Your body will start feeling less lethargic and more energised and you will have naturally started to reduce your bloating and will have likely lost a little weight.

We all need to see progress to continue a programme, so know that with every day you are making small steps forward to getting closer and closer to your goal.

I hope you all have the best day – wow DAY 9!!! Remember, we're all in this together!

DAY 10

Woohoo hello Day 10! How are you all feeling?! You're in the swing of things now and hopefully feeling the benefits as each day passes.

Take some time to reflect on how far you've come, as this is a great way to stay motivated.

Can you believe we are halfway through the programme tomorrow? This week is all about consistency and maintaining all the programme elements in a way that fits into your own personal schedule. You are establishing your new habits and putting yourself first!!

So have the best day. Drink your water, get active, eat clean and find some calm time to breathe.

As you continue your amazing journey, take some time to think about which of your menopause symptoms are easing or disappearing. Write about it in your journal and take a look back at Day 1 – can you see and feel the changes? Hopefully those cravings have subsided for you now, but if not, keeping pushing through and don't give in!

Have the best day.

DAY 11

DAY 11! You're halfway! This is such a great day as mentally you know you have not only got just 10 days to go, but that you've also been kind and good to yourself for 11 days. By now you should be feeling the benefits.

If you've managed to exercise daily, follow the nutrition guide and drink plenty of water, your body will be strengthening, you're toning up, you're eating cleanly, you're clearing your fuzzy head and headaches, your joints and body should feel less achy and bloated and you should feel like you understand yourself a little better and are starting to regain control.

I want you to feel proud of yourself and stick with it. If you've had a few blips then make today your clean eating day and definitely add a strength workout in – remember it's the strength workouts that will really help settle those hormones.

Wow girls – be proud of getting to DAY 11.

YOU'VE TOTALLY GOT THIS.

DAY 12

Hi ladies, it's DAY 12 and it's a day to celebrate your week, to feel proud of where you're at and, if your weekend is approaching, plan to make it a good one!

You got through your first weekend with determination, and this weekend you are on a roll so try and stick with it. Day 14 is a rest day from specific exercise, but again try and stay as clean as you can with your eating.

Please look back at your first day and remember why you started this programme. Look at your goals and your symptoms and take note of what positive changes you are feeling. If you've been following the programme as closely as you can you'll be really feeling the benefits of your new eating habits and exercise along with the sleep, water and self-care.

You are being kinder to yourself and learning what your body and mind needs to help you feel good.

So, plan forward like you did on week 1 make sure you have everything you need to stay on track and go into your weekend (If it's Saturday tomorrow!) with a positive 'I can do this' attitude – because you are doing this and YOU'RE WINNING.

DAY 13

Hi ladies! It may be Day 13 but there's nothing unlucky about it. Can you believe we've nearly reached two weeks on the programme? It's amazing!

Today is a great day for a strength-building workout. Pop your music on and enjoy which ever workout you choose – just 20 minutes will have you feeling strong and uplifted at the end.

Take stock today of how far you've come. You've been on this new journey for nearly two weeks – how do you feel?

Can you see some of your symptoms have lifted? Do you feel stronger? Are you feeling a little more confident? Are you starting to trust yourself and recognise what your body likes and doesn't like?

Don't forget to celebrate – and if you had a blip this week, recognise that you've got through it and you're back on track. Have a fab day – you have a rest day from exercise tomorrow. If it's the weekend for you, make sure you enjoy it. Keep drinking water, be kind to yourself, eat cleanly, move your amazing bodies and get some lovely restful sleep.

Have the best day!

DAY 14

Two weeks done! This is such a great milestone and you've smashed it.

You're on your own menopause journey and I hope those hormones are no longer dominating your day, your mind and your energy.

This coming week is all about sticking with it and pushing yourselves so you don't get complacent. It's about seeing how much better you can feel continuously.

If there's something you've resisted trying or avoided then give it a go – whether that's Priming, walking every day, drinking enough water, or a new kind of workout. See what new habits you can create to keep your journey interesting and keep seeing positive results.

This is all about getting your habits in place to carry on after the 21 days so this week will be about preparing for the rest of your menopause journey.

Start thinking about some new goals to keep you motivated. Now you're two weeks in, you'll be able to look further ahead and know that you are on the right track for feeling more like the old you – so what would she really like to do next!

Write it in your journal and keep thinking forward.

Have the best day! You've totally got this.

APPENDIX:

DAY 15

DAY 15! You are doing brilliantly.

We have six days until we get our measurements, photos and have a proper check in on our hormone symptoms.

Remember, if you have a blip day get back on it with water, walking, mindset and mindfulness, clean eating, exercise and sleep hygiene. All these combined will bring you the results you are looking for and will help you see if there is anything underlying that needs additional support when the programme is finished.

If symptoms of feeling extremely low, lethargic or tearful, are still quite prominent. Then this is when you can start to think about additional support whether it's HRT (if you're able to go on it) or getting a check up on your thyroid to see if it's out of balance.

The most important thing is to stick with it, do what you're doing and enjoy your day.

You've totally got this, have the best day.

DAY 16

Good morning, it's DAY 16!

We only have five days of the programme to go before we check in with ourselves with the fitness test, measurements, photo and hormone progress. So let's focus and really stick with what we're doing.

Make sure you're getting your strength exercises in, no matter how short! Being active each day is critical to hormone balance along with the other four elements: water, clean eating, self- care and sleep.

This should be a little mantra in your head by now. Remember to check in with yourself and take note of what you need to plan in for your day.

You are all doing so well and I really want to help you get those positive results, both mentally and physically. Focus on one thing you want to improve on this week. Is it a burpee, is it a tricep dip, is it a plank hold?! And use the next five days to strengthen yourself for that.

When you focus on something more specific than just weight loss or feelings, it will help to move you forward and achieve your goals. Have the best day.

DAY 17

Woohoo DAY 17 – let's do this!

Let's shake ourselves up, get those endorphins kicked up a notch with some energy and suppress those cortisol low mood feelings. We have four days left on this particular journey of getting to know ourselves and learning what's working.

You're doing brilliantly and will be dealing with different external pressures – but in this programme know that you are smashing it and doing something important for you.

Don't forget to look back to Day 1, look where you are today, look at those goals – reach for them again today and you'll feel great. Today you can choose your own workout and enjoy whatever movement will make you smile.

Have the best day – be strong, eat clean, drink water, find five minutes for yourself, and plan for a great sleep tonight.

You've totally got this.

DAY 18

Good Morning DAY 18 – another week is flying by. How are you feeling today?

I hope you're feeling proud, that you're keeping positive, dealing with all your life issues, whilst still eating cleanly, exercising when you can – hopefully daily – drinking that water to hydrate, clear toxins and boost head clarity, taking a little time for self-care and managing to get some quality sleep.

Only three days to go so keep pushing forward – you've totally got this.

I hope you're doing your morning Priming to get your headspace clear and positive for your day ahead – it boosts energy and helps refocus tired minds towards a positive mindset where everything is possible.

Have the best day – you've totally got this now so keep going, keep pushing forward, and keep positive.

DAY 19

Good morning my 21 Day Queens. Wow, we are on Day 19!

I hope you've had a great week and are feeling stronger, clearer headed, calmer and more in control of those lovely hormones.

Let's keep our positivity going and end on a high. Today is a great day for an arms and legs workout – you can do both or make use of what time you have and get at least one done. Tomorrow is a rest day from the exercises so make the most of today's energy blast!

Make sure you write down how you feel and where you're at – are there areas you still feel catch you out in a day? Let's try and get those targeted so the new habits you've been creating really settle in and last.

Each of us have different work/life issues which will catch us out, so you may be "choosing" certain parts of the programme to make it more manageable, or you may have had some blips.

Regardless of all that, let's make sure we smash it today and plan for the coming fitness test and photos, so the results make you smile and you can feel elated that you've reached your 21 days.

Positivity equals success.

DAY 20

Woohoo – it's Day 20 which is officially a rest day for you!

How has your week been? Can you believe you are nearly at day 21!

Tomorrow is Day 21 on this programme, the day when you'll be doing your measurements, photos and symptom reviews.

Even though today is a rest day, make sure you have a little dance around the lounge and have a good giggle. And make sure you stick with all the good things you've been doing like drinking plenty of water, walking, clean eating, self-care and good sleep. Tomorrow you'll be able to smash it and really get a sense of self-achievement.

Tomorrow, plan to get your weigh-in done first thing before you eat and drink anything. Also get your photos retaken in the same clothing as your original photos and the same position.

Please also take your measurements. I'd love you to email me your results and photos to show me how great you've done. Email hello@50shadesofmenopause.co.uk with how you feel, what symptoms have eased and an update on weight lost.

Journal about how you feel. What hormone-related issues do you have now? (If this is your time of the month, there might be a few heightened emotions and a little water retention.) How do you feel in general? What have you come to understand about yourself? What's working? And what's not?

You've done so brilliantly – as with any journey there are going to be rough roads, meanders, detours and setbacks, but with all that, you've kept pushing through.

You should feel so proud of yourself for sticking with it, especially on those tougher days where time was not on your side, when things didn't go as planned, when something happened to really throw you off course and slapped you in the face... When you have days like that, that's when you have to breathe, take stock and keep going – and you did exactly that.

So, enjoy today – it's a day to reflect and think about how you want to move forward. Are you going to join me for the my Maintenance Programme to carry on what you've been doing? Or have you mastered it so you can keep going?

Psychologically it's great to do a programme for an entire month so you can know you've been on a healthy course for that period of time. But even if you don't choose to take it any further, there's no pressure – any changes you have made as a result of following this book will have really started you on a good journey, so let's make today count.

Have the best day - you've totally got this.

DAY 21

Congratulations you've reached Day 21! That's FABU-LOUS!

Before you eat or drink anything today, stand on the scales and weigh yourself. You can also take your photo and measurements so you know where you are with those too.

Compare these to your measurements from the start of the programme to help you see how well you're doing. Remember it's ONLY been 21 days, so when you see the changes you'll be really chuffed.

Physically you will be a lot stronger. So get your fitness test done to prove it to yourself and write down your new results.

Also make sure to write down your menopause symptoms. How are you feeling? Do you have a foggy head? Are you feeling low? Do you have aching joints? Can you see how you have improved? Have you got more energy? Do you feel healthier from eating cleanly and exercising most days? You need to recognise these things so you can continue your menopause journey positively as you've taken such big steps already.

Today is about celebrating a milestone that you may not have reached on your own. You have started to form new healthier habits and have given yourself more self-care and time to breathe. You've focused on sleeping more, hydrating and drinking more water to feed your cells and clear your head, and you've cut your sugar intake which will have dramatically helped your hormonal spiral.

I hope you feel proud of yourself – you've done this along-side daily stresses and events, work pressures, maybe house renovations, or recovering from illness and you've got here! Be proud of yourself, be happy and feel how good your body is.

From here moving forward try and keep the healthier habits going so that you feed your mind and body with health and love so you can enjoy the rest of your menopause journey.

Well done you for getting 21 days done!

You're a SUPERSTAR

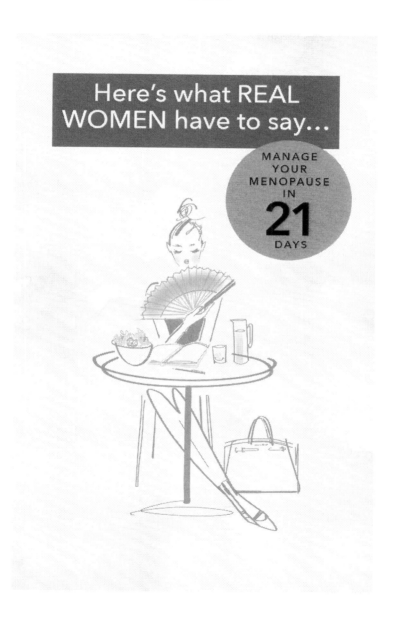

TESTIMONIALS

Here are some Testimonials from women who have completed the programme just like you

Carys started the programme in 2020, and says:

"I have finished Ailsa's 21 Day Menopause Programme and I wanted to share my experience. I am a menopausal woman who came to the programme on a background of being overweight and with poor fitness.

I have had attempts at getting fit and losing weight previously, but always gained it back and gave up. I have to admit I felt intimidated by the thought of starting this programme. There was no need!

Ailsa and this 21 Day Programme has been a life changer for me. I made the decision to commit fully for 21 days, embracing the nutritional changes and regular exercising, and the results have been amazing.

My menopause symptoms of hot flushes, feeling sluggish and de-motivated, joint pain and memory lapses have really improved

and in most cases are non-existent. I have lost several inches around my body and 13lbs in weight, which I'm really thrilled by. The advice and support that Ailsa gives is key to this programme and my success. There's no judgment here just positive messages and encouragement. Ailsa is always happy to answer any questions you may have.

The variety of exercises are brilliant and kept me motivated

… I feel lighter, brighter and more positive and I want to keep feeling this way and seeing and feeling the benefits. Ailsa, you're a star.

The group chat has been brilliant too, full of tips and lovely encouragement for each other. So if you are thinking of doing this programme my advice would be… GO FOR IT! You'll be amazed at how much better you will feel after just 21 days."

Another from Jayne, who also joined the programme in 2020:

"I have just completed the 21 Day Menopause Programme with Ailsa and for me it has been a game changer. I didn't think at the beginning of this journey I would have felt this much better after just 21 days … I don't have any of the menopausal symptoms I was experiencing – brain fog, low mood, bloating, lethargy and just generally not feeling good about myself; it has changed in just 3 weeks.

Ailsa has made me rethink my whole approach to exercise and the whole package – nutrition, mindfulness, sleep, water, meditation and body conditioning. I can't believe I am saying this but I've actually enjoyed the last 3 weeks – not something I've said *after completing any other programme. I have got so much out of the challenge and met a lovely group of like-minded ladies who have supported each other on this journey. I've also lost weight, dropped centimetres everywhere and improved my fitness plus I'm feeling healthier and happier. What more could I have wanted?*

Ailsa is one in a million. She is so supportive, loving and talented! I loved every single exercise class I participated in and the great thing is you can do them when it suits your schedule. The mix of everything is spot on and I can't recommend this programme enough – so much so I'm going on to do another 4 weeks as part of the maintenance programme.

I feel I've got myself back and that's thanks to Ailsa and this programme."

Gudrun says:

"I am so glad I found Ailsa's programme at this point in time as it really was the kick that I needed to start eating healthier again, look after myself, improve my fitness and get some energy back!

Ailsa has been so motivating and encouraging and the support of the group of women also participating was really helpful and inspiring! Ailsa is a great coach and instructor with the necessary experience that shines through.

I was concerned before I started that I might not be fit enough to keep up with the exercise routine, but Ailsa always offered options, low impact and/or modifications that even with injury I could do and am getting better!!! I have noticed a big change not only in the weight that I lost but I'm also feeling more energetic, more motivated and my body feels stronger too! The options to choose exercises at a time to suit you and have a variety of classes in style and length is great! Thanks Ailsa!"

Erica Cooke says:

"I've just completed Ailsa's 21 day kickstart programme aimed at peri-menopausal & menopausal women. It has focussed on nutrition, exercise, mindfulness & hormone re-balance. The support & guidance has been outstanding. The information, science and visual interaction has been a life changer for me (alongside my HRT). I have lost 7lbs, as well as visible inches all over my body, particularly under my bra-line front and back!!! My peri-menopausal symptoms have just about gone, I am less fatigued, less bloated, I have more stamina, my brain is less foggy, concentration improved and i have a general feeling of balance. I have met a wonderful group of like minded women and we've shared our journey.

The results are quick, in my opinion, but it does require motivation and a willingness to address bad habits, with the mindset that the principles Ailsa advocates are for life and continued good menopause health. I would highly recommend this programme to any women over 40, seeking the solution to balance. This is 5 star"

Katherine Mc Adam says:

"I'm delighted with this programme. Ailsa has an amazing and gentle way with helping us to understand what is involved in making lifetime transformations. It's so good to understand what's happening to our bodies and why, as well as HOW to make positive long term good habits.

Traditionally when I got too busy with work or life took over, I would instantly drop my healthy exercise regime, now I know that is the worst thing I could do, instead, I embrace the exercises and healthy eating as I know how much it will help me with my 'busyness'. Giving up sugar and alcohol were interesting too, because I thought that they didn't affect me much. Boy was I wrong! The first time I had alcohol for a while after giving it up I noticed a massive difference. Happy to be a 'tea totaller'. I also really like the way Ailsa shines a light on all these different areas. Keeping a spotlight on these issues ensures I keep true to my goals and am not tempted to fall off the wagon."

Lindsay Harris says:

"I am 73 and wish I had had this type of programme when I was going through my menopause. It was never a discussion that we had with anyone but a doctor and they never gave it any particular significance as 'all women go through it' and we were left feeling that we just had to get on with it. I have really benefitted hugely from this programme and feel the most alive and energised in years!

Thank you Ailsa, you are so inspirational..."

What's so great is that these amazing women are just like you and me. They reached a point where they wanted to take back some control and the results have been fantastic to see. They are all continuing with the new habits they created from doing the programme and continue to feel energised and happy.

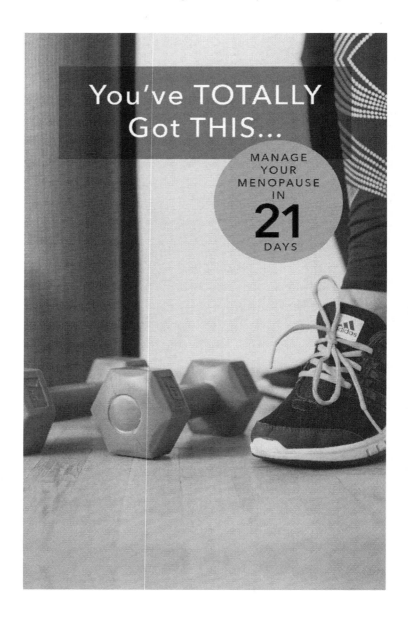

You've TOTALLY Got THIS...

MANAGE YOUR MENOPAUSE IN

21

DAYS

DISCLAIMER

Although the 21 day programme has been successful for myself and many women I am not a gynaecologist, doctor or specialist.

Every woman experiences a different combination of symptoms and so I cannot guarantee that you will achieve full easing of all your symptoms as you may require additional medical support.

However, if you follow the programme as closely as you can, you will give yourself the opportunity to feel better in several areas of your life to help you deal with the next steps you need to take.

If you already have an underlying medical condition including but not limited to, obesity, high blood pressure, diabetes, heart disease, thyroid issues, cancer or recovering from physical injury then please seek medical advice before starting any new health programme.

Your level of success in obtaining results will be dependent on many factors relating to your genetics, age, health and symptoms. I always ask you to exercise to your level of fitness and maintain the programme as best you can. Results will be slow for some and fast for others and will vary.

This is only a 21 day programme to be used as a kickstart to new healthier lifestyle habits.

Your health and wellbeing are at the forefront of why I wrote and created this book, but you will need to start getting to know yourself and your body to understand what you need to do to continue a positive menopause and post menopause life

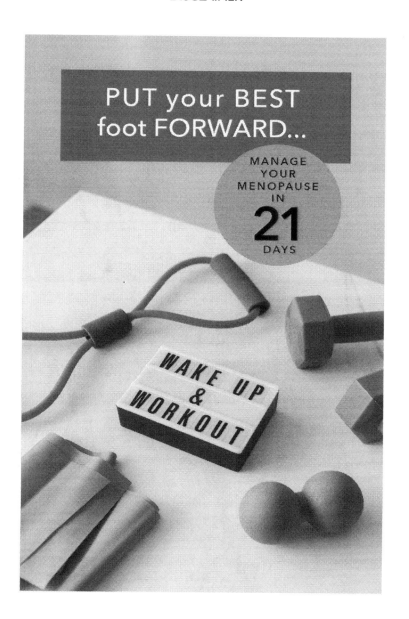

REFERENCES

1. Newson, L.R, (2021) Understanding hormone levels in the blood, My Menopause Doctor, viewed 29 March 2021. https://d2931px9t312xa. cloudfront. net/menopausedoctor/files/information/582/ Understanding %20 hormone%20levels%20in%20 the%20 blood.pdf

2. Johnson, T, (2021) 'Menopause, Weight Gain and Exercise Tips' Web M.D., viewed 30 March 2021. https: //www.webmd.com/menopause/guide/ menopause-weight-gain-and-exercise-tips

3. Waghorn, M, (2018) 'One in three UK adults not getting enough exercise, says study', Independent, viewed 30 March 2021 https://www.independent. co .uk/news/uk/home-news/uk-adults-exercise-risk-disease-exercise-world- health-organisation-a8522591 .html

4. Bansal, R & Aggarwal, N, (2019) 'Menopausal Hot Flashes: A Concise Review', Journal of Midlife Health, 2019 Jan-Mar; 10(1): 6–13, doi: 10.4103/ jmh.JMH_-7_19

REFERENCES

5. American Psychological Association. (2015). '2015 Stress in America', viewed 29 March 2021 http://www.apa.org/news/press/releases/ stress/2015/snapshot.aspx

6. NHS UK, (2021) 'Hormone Replacement Therapy', viewed 21 April 2021 https://www.nhs.uk/conditions/hormone-replacement-therapy-hrt/

7. Premier Health, (2017) 'Consider Pros and Cons of Hormone Replacement Therapy', viewed 30 March 2021 https://www.premierhealth. com/your-health/articles/women%27s-health-update/consider-pros-and- cons-of-hormone-replacement-therapy

8. Mason, J.K, Thompson, L.U,(2014) 'Flaxseed and its lignan and oil components: can they play a role in reducing the risk of an improving the treatment of breast cancer?', Appl Physiol Nutr Metab, 2014 Jun;39(6):663-78. doi: 10.1139/apnm-2013-0420

9. Gentry-Maharaj A, Karpinskyj C, Glazer C, et al. Use and perceived efficacy of complementary and alternative medicines after discontinuation of hormone therapy: a nested United Kingdom Collaborative Trial of Ovarian Cancer Screening cohort study. Menopause. 2015;22(4):384-390. doi:10.1097/GME.0000000000000330

10. Rani, A, Anupam S. "The genus Vitex: A review." Pharmacognosy reviews vol. 7,14 (2013): 188-98. doi:10.4103/0973-7847.120522

11. Ghazanfarpour M, Sadeghi R, Latifnejad Roudsari R, et al. 'Effects of red clover on hot flash and circulating hormone concentrations in menopausal women: a systematic review and meta-analysis.' Avicenna J Phytomed. 2015;5(6):498-511.

12. Rani, A, Anupam S. "The genus Vitex: A review." Pharmacognosy reviews vol. 7,14 (2013): 188-98. doi:10.4103/0973-7847.120522

13. Stover PJ. 'Vitamin B12 and older adults'. Curr Opin Clin Nutr Metab Care. 2010;13(1):24-27. doi:10.1097 /MCO.0b013e328333 d157

14. Yang Q, Zhang Z, Gregg EW, Flanders WD, Merritt R, Hu FB. 'Added sugar intake and cardiovascular diseases mortality among US adults.' JAMA Intern Med. 2014 Apr;174(4):516-24. doi: 10.1001/jamainternmed.2013.13563. PMID: 24493081.

15. Yang Q, Zhang Z, Gregg EW, Flanders WD, Merritt R, Hu FB. 'Added sugar intake and cardiovascular diseases mortality among US adults.' JAMA Intern Med. 2014 Apr;174(4):516-24. doi: 10.1001/jamainternmed.2013.13563. PMID: 24493081.

16. Kucharska A, Szmurło A, Si⊠ska B. Significance of diet in treated and untreated acne vulgaris. Postepy Dermatol Alergol. 2016;33(2):81-86. doi:10.5114/ada.2016.59146

17. Gkogkolou P, Böhm M. Advanced glycation end products: Key players in skin aging?. Dermatoendocrinol. 2012;4(3):259-270. doi:10.4161/ derm.22028

REFERENCES

18. Leung, CW, Laraia B.A, et al (2015) 'Soda and Cell Aging: Associations Between Sugar-Sweetened Beverage Consumption and Leukocyte Telomere Length in Healthy Adults From the National Health and Nutrition Surveys', American Journal of Public Health, 2014 December; 104(12): 2425–2431 doi: 10.2105/AJPH .2014.302151

19. Beilharz JE, Maniam J, Morris MJ. Short-term exposure to a diet high in fat and sugar, or liquid sugar, selectively impairs hippocampal-dependent memory, with differential impacts on inflammation. Behav Brain Res. 2016;306:1-7. doi:10.1016/j.bbr.2016.03.018

20. Beilharz JE, Maniam J, Morris MJ. Diet-Induced Cognitive Deficits: The Role of Fat and Sugar, Potential Mechanisms and Nutritional Interventions. Nutrients. 2015;7(8):6719-6738. doi:10.3390/nu7085307

21. Cirino, E, (2020) 'Chewing Your Food: Is 32 Really the Magic Number?' Healthline, viewed 30 March 2021 https://www.healthline.com/health/how- many-times-should-you-chew-your-food

22. Luppino FS, de Wit LM, Bouvy PF, Stijnen T, Cuijpers P, Penninx BW, Zitman FG, (2010) 'Overweight, obesity, and depression: a systematic review and meta-analysis of longitudinal studies'.Arch Gen Psychiatry. 2010 Mar; 67(3):220-9.

23. He Q, Xiao L, Xue G, et al. 'Poor ability to resist tempting calorie rich food is linked to altered balance

between neural systems involved in urge and self-control.' Nutr J. 2014;13:92. Published 2014 Sep 16. doi:10.1186/1475-2891-13-92

24. Binu, S, (2019) 'Here's why you should eat at the same time every day', Netmeds, viewed 30 March 2021 https://www.netmeds.com/health-library/ post/ here-s-why-you-should-eat-at-same-time-every-day

25. Mills S, Brown H, Wrieden W, White M, Adams J. 'Frequency of eating home cooked meals and potential benefits for diet and health: cross- sectional analysis of a population-based cohort study.' Int J Behav Nutr Phys Act. 2017;14(1):109. Published 2017 Aug 17. doi:10.1186/s12966-017-0567-y

26. Chang T, Ravi N, Plegue MA, Sonneville KR, Davis MM. Inadequate Hydration, BMI, and Obesity Among US Adults: NHANES 2009-2012. Ann Fam Med. 2016;14(4):320-324. doi:10.1370/afm.1951

27. Dennis EA, Dengo AL, Comber DL, Flack KD, Savla J, Davy KP, Davy BM. 'Water consumption increases weight loss during a hypocaloric diet intervention in middle-aged and older adults.' Obesity (Silver Spring). 2010 Feb;18(2):300-7. doi: 10.1038/oby.2009.235. Epub 2009 Aug 6. PMID: 19661958; PMCID: PMC 2859815.

28. Rachel Homes – Fitness Instructor, Online Health, Fitness, Wellness and education provider for Fitness Professionals.

About the Author

Ailsa Petchey is a mother of two, wife and entrepreneur. She loves personal fitness, wellbeing, photography and spending her relaxation time with family and friends.

Ailsa has previously written and co-authored a bridal book '21st Century Bride' and 'The Complete Wedding Guide' for Marks & Spencer, published by Time Warner, whilst she was director at Virgin Brides in London.

Throughout she has maintained her love of fitness and instruction and when affected by her own menopause experiences, knew she had to write this book to share ways to help others going through their own journey.

'One day at a time' and 'you've totally got this' are her daily mantra's, to pick herself up and tackle each day head on.

'We are all unique and we will have our own menopause experience, but I hope this book will support, guide and inspire women to find a positive path and know they're not alone'.

Printed in Great Britain
by Amazon